Have Great Sex

This book is dedicated to Smithy who has tested everything with me and I hope always will.

Teach® Yourself

Have Great Sex
Paul Jenner

For UK order enquiries: please contact Bookpoint Ltd, 130 Milton Park, Abingdon, Oxon OX14 4SB. Telephone: +44 (0) 1235 827720. Fax: +44 (0) 1235 400454. Lines are open 09.00–17.00, Monday to Saturday, with a 24-hour message answering service. Details about our titles and how to order are available at www.teachyourself.com

For USA order enquiries: please contact McGraw-Hill Customer Services, PO Box 545, Blacklick, OH 43004-0545, USA. Telephone: 1-800-722-4726. Fax: 1-614-755-5645.

For Canada order enquiries: please contact McGraw-Hill Ryerson Ltd, 300 Water St, Whitby, Ontario L1N 9B6, Canada. Telephone: 905 430 5000. Fax: 905 430 5020.

Long renowned as the authoritative source for self-guided learning – with more than 50 million copies sold worldwide – the **Teach Yourself** series includes over 500 titles in the fields of languages, crafts, hobbies, business, computing and education.

British Library Cataloguing in Publication Data: a catalogue record for this title is available from the British Library.

Library of Congress Catalog Card Number: on file.

First published in UK 2006 by Hodder Education, part of Hachette UK, 338 Euston Road, London NW1 3BH.

First published in US 2006 by The McGraw-Hill Companies, Inc.

This edition published 2010.

Previously published as *Teach Yourself Great Sex*

The **Teach Yourself** name is a registered trade mark of Hodder Headline.

Typeset by MPS Limited, a Macmillan Company.

Printed in Great Britain for Hodder Education, an Hachette UK Company, 338 Euston Road, London NW1 3BH, by CPI Cox & Wyman, Reading, Berkshire RG1 8EX.

The publisher has used its best endeavours to ensure that the URLs for external websites referred to in this book are correct and active at the time of going to press. However, the publisher and the author have no responsibility for the websites and can make no guarantee that a site will remain live or that the content will remain relevant, decent or appropriate.

Hachette UK's policy is to use papers that are natural, renewable and recyclable products and made from wood grown in sustainable forests. The logging and manufacturing processes are expected to conform to the environmental regulations of the country of origin.

Impression number   10 9 8 7 6 5 4 3 2 1

Year   2014 2013 2012 2011 2010

Acknowledgements

A very special thank you to Richard Craze; to Victoria Roddam, my publisher at Hodder Education; to Katie Archer and Laura Davis at Hodder Education; to my editor, Althea Brooks; and to all those who took part in my focus groups.

Contents

Meet the author

My mission in this book is not only to increase the sexual pleasure you give one another, and derive from one another, but also to encourage you to have sex far more often, for far longer and in a far more varied way.

Surveys suggest that the average young couple makes love three times a week for just a few minutes, and that frequency tapers off as the years go by. Also, my own experience within focus groups I have run is that most people still feel a lot of guilt about sex. My aim is to change that.

This, then, is an extraordinary situation. For all the talk of living in a highly sexualized society, the reality is that most couples spend far more time on just about everything and anything else, than on having sex.

What is great sex? Great sex is physical, emotional, intellectual and spiritual. Great sex:

▶ *lasts at least an hour from start to finish*
▶ *takes you to the very limits of physical pleasure*
▶ *is emotionally reinforcing*
▶ *awakens your spirituality*
▶ *gives you orgasms in your mind as well as in your body*
▶ *uncovers things about yourself and your partner that you didn't know before.*

This book will tell you almost everything you need to know about the physical aspects of sex, from the ancient wisdom of the Tao right up to the latest discoveries about male multiple orgasms and female ejaculation. I deliberately say 'almost everything' because, no matter how much you study technique, there's always something special that has to come from you – something unique, something only *you* can give. Apart from that, nobody can ever know everything about sex. That's one of the things that makes it so wonderful. No matter how much experience you have, there are always new things to discover.

Where *Have Great Sex* differs from so many other manuals is in its equal emphasis on the *psychological* aspects of sex as well as the physical aspects. The key to great sex with a partner is great communication. Two people will never have great sex with one another if they don't understand one another's bodies, responses, characters, inhibitions and emotional needs. And this is not easy because very few people even know themselves well, let alone understand a partner, especially a partner of the opposite sex.

This book is aimed primarily at heterosexual couples in long-term relationships, but there's plenty here that equally applies to same-sex couples, and much that can be adapted. If you're at a stage of your life when you're unsure of your sexual orientation, the information and ideas in this book may provide the basis for experimentation.

Is it possible to have better sex with a partner if only one of you reads this book? The answer is emphatically 'yes'. There's a great deal you can do to make sex better for both of you by working not just on your technique but on your whole approach to sex and, indeed, your relationship. Sex with another person is about giving not taking, and it only takes one person to give. It's so often the case that what you perceive as your partner's problem is really *your* problem. But, of course, try to get your partner to read the book as well. You'll find questionnaires and self-tests that you can both complete so that you can compare answers afterwards. Almost certainly you will discover things about one another that will surprise you.

With a book such as this, there's always the impulse to open it at techniques and positions and to 'get on with it', and there's no reason why you can't. Yet if you do that, I'd recommend that later you turn to the beginning and read through the book in order. If you miss some chapters out, you might not understand how certain techniques work or can even be possible. For the same reason, don't just concentrate on the practical exercises but read the background explanations as well. It's only once you understand how bodies work that you can go on to improvise your own techniques.

WHAT DOES GREAT SEX MEAN TO YOU?

Tick the things that constitute great sex to you right now. After you've followed the advice in this book, see if you still agree.

- ☐ I will have sex more often.
- ☐ I will have more sex partners.
- ☐ I will have more orgasms.
- ☐ I will experiment with more positions and techniques.
- ☐ I will use sex toys.
- ☐ I will do the things I've always wanted to do but never dared.
- ☐ I will not hold anything back.
- ☐ I will feel completely uninhibited.
- ☐ I will feel completely loved.
- ☐ I will feel more satisfied at the end of sex.
- ☐ I will give my partner more orgasms.
- ☐ I will have more empathy with my partner.
- ☐ I will know I have completely satisfied my partner.
- ☐ I will feel a spiritual connection with my lover.
- ☐ I will feel a spiritual connection with the whole universe.

Nothing else comes remotely close to sex in terms of the ecstasy one person can create in another. So right now, resolve to set aside plenty of time for sex. Long sex sessions aren't automatically great but great sex sessions are always long. Have plenty of them.

Only got a minute?

Good sex is possible with someone you like but great sex is only possible with someone you love. Here is a quick summary of tips you'll find in the book.

- Masturbate regularly to explore your own body and practise techniques – and watch one another masturbate.
- Don't make sex routine but have some sort of sex routinely – ideally every day.
- Quickies can be nice but for great sex set aside at least an hour – create the right atmosphere with a shared shower, music, incense and romantic lighting.
- Great communication is vital for great sex.
- Only a third of women orgasm from vaginal stimulation alone – always include the clitoris.
- In addition to the usual places, try the clitoral glans (by gently retracting the hood), the G-spot, the anal canal, the prostate and the tongue.

- Try artificial lubricant.
- Work through the 35 great sex positions and 32 variations in this book and you'll get to know one another very well.
- Your mind is actually your most important sex organ – stimulate it with shared sexual fantasies.
- Multiple orgasms are for women *and* men.
- Sex without ejaculation avoids the refractory period and the 'sexual hangover'.
- For twenty-first century sex, try a few twenty-first century sex toys.
- Pay attention to the post-orgasmic period.
- Increase 'sex chemicals' by doing 'sexercises'.
- Give your sex drive a boost with erotica and food supplements such as Maca and Ginkgo biloba.

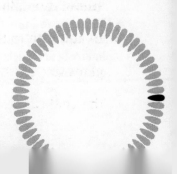

5 Only got five minutes?

1 A great attitude to sex

▶ The things that make a good sex life great are open communication, freedom from guilt, frequent lovemaking... and love itself.

2 Women's bodies

▶ There are at least 11 good reasons to masturbate frequently – don't feel guilty about it.
▶ Only one-third of women can orgasm from intercourse alone – clitoral stimulation is vital.
▶ The G-spot *does* exist and women *can* ejaculate.
▶ Switching between clitoral and G-spot stimulation prolongs orgasm.

3 Men's bodies

▶ There are at least 12 good reasons to masturbate frequently (but not necessarily to ejaculate) – don't feel guilty about it.
▶ The anus and prostate are also sources of pleasure.
▶ Orgasm and ejaculation are not the same thing; prolonging intercourse by delaying ejaculation is one of the keys to great sex.

4 Great opening moves

▶ Keep the sexual temperature up all the time in your relationship, through body language, sexy emails and texts, cuddling and massage.

5 Great sex techniques

▶ Spend at least an hour stimulating every part of one another's bodies and your own bodies including the anal areas, the G-spot and the prostate.
▶ If you're finding it difficult to orgasm simultaneously, a trick to make a woman come quickly is for her to masturbate during intercourse; a trick to make a man come quickly is to insert a finger into his anus.

6 Great positions

▶ Different positions create different physical and psychological effects, as well as providing variety – in this book you'll find 35 main positions and 32 variations.

7 Great sex is in the mind

▶ Your most important sex organ lies not between your thighs but between your ears. Use visualization, 'talking dirty' and shared fantasies as ways of raising the sexual temperature.

8 Great multiple orgasms

▶ A vibrator will help any woman become multi-orgasmic – vibrators and artificial lubricant are probably the two greatest 'sex toys'.

▶ Men can also enjoy multiple orgasms (but without ejaculation) leading to higher levels of excitement.

9 Great toys, tricks and aphrodisiacs

▶ Extra excitement can be created by bondage (but only with someone you know *very* well), a slap along with the tickle, a shaven vulva, a mirror and an erotic film.

10 After orgasm

▶ Romantic music, cuddles, shared food and drink, and non-ejaculation (by a man) all help prolong that loving mood.

11 Fitness for great sex

▶ The fitter you are, the slimmer you are, the less saturated fat you eat, the less you smoke and drink alcohol, the better your sexual performance.

12 Great sex during and after pregnancy

▶ Intercourse is safe at all stages of a pregnancy that has no complications but most women feel like it only during months four to seven; the six weeks after birth (when sex isn't possible) are a great time for men to refine their multi-orgasmic technique.

13 Great sex ever after

▶ Sex can go on getting better and better almost indefinitely, provided you keep doing it regularly (even daily) and practise your technique.

14 Great solutions to some common sex problems

▶ There are simple solutions to most sexual problems, provided you can talk about them calmly, openly and without guilt.

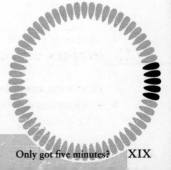

10 Only got ten minutes?

1 A great attitude to sex

- Being in love doesn't guarantee great sex, but you're even less likely to experience great sex if you're not in love.
- Good communication equals good sex, and bad communication equals bad sex; if you feel guilty about your body you'll never enjoy great sex.
- Make sex a regular part of your relationship – don't wait until you're 'desperate'.

2 Women's bodies

- There are at least 11 good reasons to masturbate frequently – don't feel guilty about it.
- The clitoris is just the tip of a much larger organ which is analogous to the penis.
- Only one-third of women can orgasm from intercourse alone.
- The G-spot *does* exist and women *can* ejaculate.
- Orgasms can be intensified by strengthening the PC muscle, and by switching between clitoral and G-spot stimulation.

3 Men's bodies

- There are at least 12 good reasons to masturbate frequently (but not necessarily to ejaculate) – don't feel guilty about it.
- Pleasure isn't related to penis size but to technique; pleasure can be increased by also stimulating the anus and the prostate.
- Orgasm and ejaculation can be intensified by strengthening the PC muscle.

- Orgasm and ejaculation are not the same thing; prolonging intercourse by delaying ejaculation is one of the keys to great sex.
- The locking method, which helps prevent ejaculation, involves contracting the PC and abdominal muscles simultaneously.

---

4 Great opening moves

- Keep the sexual temperature up all the time in your relationship, through body language, sexy emails and texts, cuddling and massage.
- For great sex establish the mood with lighting, music and scent.
- Reliable contraceptive methods that don't interfere with pleasure include the pill, vasectomy, female sterilization, the patch, the implant, the injection and the IUS; for young couples, condoms can actually increase pleasure by prolonging intercourse.

---

5 Great sex techniques

- One hour is the minimum for great sex.
- Show one another how you masturbate and enjoy doing it together.
- Stimulate the entire skin surface; on a woman's body pay particular attention to her neck, ears, nipples, areolas and breasts.
- Tell your partner exactly how you like cunnilingus/fellatio done.
- Include the anal area in sex play.
- Use pressure and a gentle 'come here' movement on the G-spot.
- If you're finding it difficult to orgasm simultaneously, a trick to make a woman come quickly is for her to masturbate

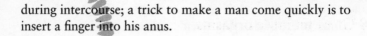

during intercourse; a trick to make a man come quickly is to insert a finger into his anus.

6 Great positions

▶ There are 35 positions in this chapter, plus 32 variations, and you should try them all, although most of the time you'll probably just stick with half a dozen.

▶ The *Missionary* can be improved by a cushion under the buttocks for easier cunnilingus and to enable the man to squat and move more freely.

▶ From the *Improved missionary*, it's easy for a woman to roll back into a *Ball* or to become an *Exhibitionist* by swinging her open legs back over her head.

▶ The *Rider*, in which the woman lies face down on the bed and the man sits on her buttocks and upper thighs, is great for vivid G-spot stimulation.

▶ The *Sitting embrace* is a position of equality in which you can share fantasies, food and drink.

▶ *Cuddly bears*, with the woman kneeling and her face on a pillow, is a great position for anal sex.

▶ It can be fun to try switching positions without disengaging.

7 Great sex is in the mind

▶ Your most important sex organ lies not between your thighs but between your ears.

▶ The changes that sex brings about in your brain can be intensified through the power of your mind.

▶ If you're anxious about sex, put yourself in the 'zone' by visualizing success.

▶ 'Talking dirty' will raise the sexual temperature; shared fantasies can raise it even more.

8 Great multiple orgasms

- ▶ Most women can learn to experience multiple orgasms through uninhibited masturbation, especially using fantasy and a vibrator.
- ▶ Women tend to have multiple orgasms more easily as they get older, providing they have regular sex alone or with a partner.
- ▶ Men can also enjoy multiple orgasms, although they're essentially partial orgasms without ejaculation.
- ▶ Non-ejaculatory sex can build excitement to a level far beyond 'normal' sex.

9 Great toys, tricks and aphrodisiacs

- ▶ Vibrators and artificial lubricant are probably the two greatest 'sex toys'.
- ▶ Bondage provides the opportunity for one of you to really lie back and enjoy it (but only with someone you know *very* well).
- ▶ A slap along with the tickle can be very arousing (as long as it's not too hard).
- ▶ For most men, a shaven or waxed vulva is about as powerful an aphrodisiac as exists.
- ▶ Other supercharged aphrodisiacs include a mirror and an erotic film (which could be one you make of yourselves).

10 After orgasm

- ▶ Listening to romantic music while sharing food, drink and cuddles is a good way of coming down gently.
- ▶ The Coolidge Effect is part of the sexual hangover that, paradoxically, can make some men irritable after sex; sex without ejaculation is the solution.

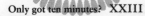

11 Fitness for great sex

- The fitter you are generally, the fitter you'll be for sex.
- Healthy food helps you to enjoy a healthy sex life.
- Foods high in saturated fats can lower testosterone and cause long-term damage to blood circulation in the genitals.
- For great sex keep your body mass index (BMI) at 24 or less.
- Working out with weights or a weight machine will give you a beautiful body; giving your PC muscle a regular workout will give you a beautiful penis/vagina.
- Smoking and too much alcohol will damage sexual performance.

12 Great sex during and after pregnancy

- Intercourse is safe at all stages of a normal pregnancy, but a doctor may tell you to stop if there are complications.
- During the first three months of pregnancy 'first-timers' generally don't feel much like sex, but women who've been pregnant before usually maintain their libidos.
- During the following four months most pregnant women feel more like sex than ever.
- The two months prior to the birth, and the six weeks after (when sex isn't possible), are a great time for men to refine their multi-orgasmic technique.

13 Great sex ever after

- Sex can go on getting better and better almost indefinitely.
- Every woman over 50 should have a vibrator, plenty of lubricant and frequent sex.
- Every man over 50 should have some erotica and masturbate regularly, but not to ejaculation.
- Daily sex is still possible for older couples who practise sex without ejaculation.

14 Great solutions to some common sex problems

▶ Good communication, in a calm atmosphere, is the key to solving disagreements about sex.
▶ A small penis is rarely a problem but, if you're concerned, jelqing (massage) may increase size without surgery.
▶ Erectile dysfunction can often be helped by removing the pressure to ejaculate – get comfortable masturbating in front of one another.

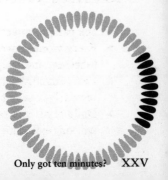

1

A great attitude to sex

In this chapter you will learn:
- *how to overcome inhibitions*
- *how sexually compatible you and your partner are*
- *how your attitude to life affects your sex life too.*

If you want to improve your sex life and enjoy great sex, you're probably thinking in terms of physical techniques. However, in fact, vital as they are, physical techniques are only part of the story. The *psychological* aspects of sex are at least as important. All the skills that are known will never turn sex into great sex unless both partners have the right mental attitudes. So don't skip this chapter in order to get on to the physical side of things as it could be by far the most important one.

Be in love

Being in love doesn't guarantee great sex, but you're even less likely to experience great sex if you're not in love. Great sex requires complicity. It requires you to find every aspect of your partner's body delightful. You need to dissolve into your partner's body and disappear. It is very unlikely that you will achieve the necessary empathy with someone you don't know very well or that you don't care about.

Be uninhibited

Try not to look at consenting sexual practices in moral terms (if you do). If you get pleasure from a part of your body that someone taught you was 'bad', accept the pleasure gratefully and don't try to hide your pleasure from your partner. If you feel guilty about your body, you'll never enjoy great sex.

It can take a long time to 'unlearn' negative feelings. A lifetime, in some cases. Here's a little test to check how you're doing.

HOW SEXUALLY INHIBITED ARE YOU?

Tick the statements you agree with.

1 *I'm quite comfortable undressing in front of my partner.* ☐
2 *I enjoy being naked on a nude beach.* ☐
3 *I think my naked body is beautiful and I like to show it.* ☐
4 *I never wear anything in bed.* ☐
5 *I like to bath/shower together with my partner.* ☐
6 *I find it easy to talk about sex with my partner.* ☐
7 *I tell my partner exactly what I want.* ☐
8 *I prefer to make love with the lights on and with the covers thrown back.* ☐
9 *I like to make love in different places.* ☐
10 *I'm not embarrassed about people knowing I masturbate.* ☐
11 *I sometimes like to masturbate or have sex in front of a mirror.* ☐
12 *I masturbate in front of my partner.* ☐
13 *I like to talk dirty during sex.* ☐
14 *I like to talk through my fantasies while having sex.* ☐
15 *I find it exciting to take photographs/make a video while having sex.* ☐
16 *I like to try new sex techniques.* ☐
17 *I'm not at all bothered about my partner seeing my face when I orgasm.* ☐

18 *I make a lot of noise when I orgasm.* ☐
19 *I think my genitals are attractive and am happy for my
    partner to see them.* ☐
20 *I think my anus is attractive and am happy for my
    partner to see it.* ☐

How did you score?

> ▶ *If you're reading this book, it's unlikely that you have fewer
>   than five ticks but if you do, you certainly need to work on your
>   inhibitions. You may find that you need some professional help,
>   especially if you have issues to do with some earlier trauma;
>   see 'Taking it further' for resources that might help you.*
> ▶ *If you scored six to ten ticks, you're still quite inhibited but
>   can probably improve with the help of this book alone.*
> ▶ *If you scored 11 to 15 ticks, you're fairly uninhibited and
>   can easily become more so.*
> ▶ *If you scored over 15 ticks, you're already extremely
>   uninhibited and will have no problem adopting the
>   suggestions in this book.*

You (and your partner, if you have one) will as a matter of course
almost certainly become less inhibited as you get older, but if you
are inhibited that's not much consolation right now. Becoming less
inhibited is not something you can just decide to do, although a
positive attitude helps. Even if you're eager to become less inhibited,
it's quite possible that your partner might find the idea frightening.

If either of you is anxious about the idea of becoming less inhibited,
it's important to understand that this does not mean doing things
you don't want to do. Nor, as some people imagine, does being
uninhibited mean ignoring the consequences of your actions and
doing whatever you feel like at that moment. It means doing things
you do really want to do but that you are afraid to do, in some
way or another, perhaps because of a subconscious block, because
of the way you were brought up or educated, because of your
self-image, or because you fear your partner's reaction.

Most people gain confidence from knowing what other people do sexually, and in 'Taking it further' you'll find a list of books that will tell you. Right now, it may help you to remember, for example, that almost all men and the vast majority of women masturbate. It may also help to know that most indulge in oral sex. It might be useful to read sexy novels and magazines and to watch erotic films.

Insight

Try to discuss sex with your close friends. Most people enjoy talking about sex, and among your friends there's bound to be somebody more open and frank than you are. (However, don't talk specifically about your partner unless he or she has given permission.)

Defining your inhibitions more precisely may be of benefit. Write a list of the things that you would like to do but that you feel you can't. Go through them one by one. Are they really so difficult? Try to visualize doing them. Break them down into easy steps. Visualize each of the steps until you get to the point that makes you worried. Repeat this over a period of time until you can visualize the action to the very end. For a more detailed explanation of this technique see Chapter 7.

Try to discuss your list with your partner. He or she will almost certainly welcome the opportunity to help solve your problems and, quite possibly, will be equally eager to discuss his or her own inhibitions at the same time.

Insight

Never wear pyjamas or nightdresses. Lovers sleep naked. If your bedroom and bed aren't warm enough then do something about it. When you wake in the night and feel lonely or anxious you want to be able to reach out and touch flesh not winceyette. Wearing clothes in bed is as silly as wearing clothes in the bath. What's more, it's a rejection of your partner. Clothes mean 'don't touch'. Naked means intimacy.

Be compatible

It's very difficult to have great sex if both of you want to dominate things or if one of you likes to try everything new and the other likes to feel safe with the familiar, or if one of you wants sex every day and the other only wants sex once a week (see 'Be frequent', page 11). In other words, it's going to be difficult to have great sex if you're not sexually compatible. So are you? If you're not sure, try this test.

HOW SEXUALLY COMPATIBLE ARE YOU?

Answer the following questions honestly and ask your partner (quite separately) to do the same.

1 *Do you regard sex as:*
 (a) *something you have to put up with?*
 (b) *something you do to please your partner?*
 (c) *a way of demonstrating love?*
 (d) *something pleasant but overrated?*
 (e) *a thrilling adventure to be explored to the limits?*

2 *I like to have sex:*
 (a) *once a week.*
 (b) *two to three times a week.*
 (c) *every two days.*
 (d) *every day.*
 (e) *more than once a day.*

3 *I think the amount of sex I have with my partner is:*
 (a) *too little.*
 (b) *about right.*
 (c) *too much.*

4 *In sex I feel:*
 (a) *my partner dominates me.*
 (b) *equal with my partner.*
 (c) *I dominate my partner.*

5 *Normally:*
    (a) *it's my partner who initiates sex.*
    (b) *we both equally initiate sex.*
    (c) *I initiate sex.*

6 *I turn down my partner's request for sex:*
    (a) *often.*
    (b) *sometimes.*
    (c) *rarely.*
    (d) *never.*

7 *My partner turns down my request for sex:*
    (a) *often.*
    (b) *sometimes.*
    (c) *rarely.*
    (d) *never.*

8 *I:*
    (a) *am happy to stick with the things we do now.*
    (b) *like trying different things.*

9 *It's normally:*
    (a) *my partner who suggests new things.*
    (b) *me who suggests new things.*

10 *I feel:*
    (a) *I'm not going to do anything special to please my partner because my partner never does anything to please me.*
    (b) *I'm always doing things to please my partner even though my partner never does anything to please me.*
    (c) *my partner is always trying to please me and I try to do the same.*

11 *I think:*
    (a) *sex is just an incidental part of a good relationship.*
    (b) *sex is a fundamental part of a good relationship.*

Were there any surprises there? Was your view of yourself the same as your partner's view of you? How did your view of your partner coincide with his or her view? Most important of all, were your views compatible?

If it seems that you're not very compatible sexually, don't despair. I said it would be difficult to have great sex, but it's not impossible. If you're in love with somebody, that's a commitment for the long haul. Attitudes can change on both sides. Don't be impatient; concentrate, first of all, on the aspects of lovemaking you *do* agree on. Enjoy them. There's nothing to say that an orgasm hanging upside down from a chandelier is any better than an orgasm in bed in the missionary position.

Insight

Compatibility doesn't mean being alike in every respect. For some things, it actually helps to be different. A person who likes to dominate will be most compatible with a partner who likes to be dominated, and many couples are perfectly happy with one initiating sex and the other following.

The real value of an exercise like this is in provoking discussion. When differences are out in the open, there's a chance of doing something about them. Once it's clear what you do and don't agree on, you can start working on possible solutions. How? Through *communication*.

Be communicative (and conciliatory)

Good communication equals good sex. Bad communication equals bad sex. It's as straightforward as that. If you want great sex, aim for great communication. In one study, 88 per cent of women who 'always' discussed their sexual feelings with their husbands said their sex lives were 'very good' or 'good'. The figure for those who 'often' discussed their sexual feelings was 80 per cent. Yet among those who only 'occasionally' discussed their sexual feelings, only 58 per cent enjoyed sex that was 'very good' or 'good'. For those who never discussed their feelings, the figure was just 30 per cent.

Good communication is really not difficult, but there is a right way and a wrong way to go about it. If there's something you're not happy about, *don't* criticize. Try to approach problems in a positive manner. For example, don't say: 'You always orgasm too soon.' Turn it around and say: 'When you manage to hold off it really drives me wild.' Everybody responds to encouragement. Criticism makes people either withdraw or attack in turn.

Of course, it's easy to be communicative when you're saying something the other person wants to hear. However, what happens when one person wants to try something and the other doesn't? Typically, somebody reads about something in a magazine or book, or sees something in a pornographic film, and wants his or her partner to emulate it. This can create one of the most difficult sexual problems in a relationship. The thing is that some people like to experiment. It's their nature. They like taking things apart to see how they work, getting to the tops of mountains and trying out whatever is new. Others, by contrast, tend to like safety, security and normality. If they're happy with what they're doing now, they don't feel the compulsion to seek new thrills to add to the repertoire.

There is an established three-part formula for these delicate occasions. First, you acknowledge the other person's feelings. Second, you state your own feelings. Third, you try to offer a positive way forward. Everyone, after all, likes to feel that their own needs are being considered and that their own ideas are being accepted as valid. For example:

Part one: 'I know you'd like me to try some particular new sex positions...'

Part two: '...but I'd find those positions very embarrassing.'

Part three: 'As a compromise, I'd be willing to try the such-and-such position if it's in the dark.'

Or:

Part one: 'I know you find certain sex positions very embarrassing...'

Part two: 'But I've already seen you naked from every angle and I love every bit of you.'

Part three: 'As a compromise, would you be willing to try the such-and-such position if it's in the dark?'

Insight

Bear in mind that your partner's, and your own, attitudes will change over time. With a considerate partner you may come to enjoy things you never thought you would. Indeed, you may not even know what your own response will be when you actually do something. You may think you know and yet when you actually experience it you may feel differently. We all have to experiment, and this is one of the things that makes sex so endlessly fascinating.

So, let's start communicating. Let's get intimate. You may be holding back because you feel you want to remain 'mysterious'. In fact, every revelation you make will simply raise more questions. The more you reveal, the more mysterious you are.

Men receive a particularly bad press when it comes to communication. There's a misconception that they're not willing to talk about things but this is not really true. What is true is that men hate criticism even more than women do because it makes them feel less like men. Most men are very insecure about their masculinity. The process of communication has to be pleasurable not painful.

It takes two to communicate so I'm hoping that you are both going to take part in the following exercise to get sexual communication going. If not though, maybe you could take a clear lead and your partner will start to get the idea.

There are all kinds of additional possibilities for provoking sexual discussion such as films with erotic content, books (including this one) and sexy board games. So get talking. But remember, we all move by small steps. Be patient and you'll be amazed how far you can go.

Be willing and active

Most of us feel pretty vulnerable when it comes to sex, and so having an invitation to sex rejected can feel extremely crushing. Try not to turn down your partner's overtures. If it happens too often, your partner may never try to initiate sex again.

Of course, we all have the right to refuse sex when we don't want it. There could be valid reasons such as fear of pregnancy, fear of impotence, and yes, even a headache. Yet when you turn down sex for yourself, you also turn down sex for your partner, so think twice. Your partner, after all, is only inviting you to take part in one of the most marvellous experiences life has to offer.

Insight

Don't adopt an 'all right, if you insist' type of attitude. That's just as upsetting as saying 'no'. If you're going to do something, you may as well do it with good grace, not to mention enthusiasm.

If you're a woman, don't be backwards in showing enthusiasm because you think it might be unfeminine – take an active role some of the time. Some men feel threatened when women take control, but that's rare nowadays. Most men will be excited and, of course, by taking equal responsibility you can guarantee your own satisfaction, just as men do.

Insight

If you have a pet dog or cat, you probably stroke it every time you pass. You probably say nice things, such as: 'He's a lovely boy.' Do you do the same for your partner? People need physical affection just as much as cats and dogs do. Whenever you pass your lover in the kitchen or on the stairs, make sure you touch. When you wake up in the morning (naked), the first thing you should do is cuddle. When you go to bed at night (naked), the last thing you should do is cuddle. And, in between, cuddle as much as possible.

Be frequent

Sex every day keeps the doctors and lawyers away.

One of the world's great mysteries is why human beings spend so much time thinking about sex, reading about sex, and watching recordings of other people having sex and yet spend so little time actually doing it themselves. The average is something like once every third day for a few minutes – maybe an hour a week. Compare that with the amount of time devoted to food. Or shopping. Or watching television.

How frequently could you have sex? The famous American researcher Alfred Kinsey found young couples who were having intercourse up to 29 times a week, that is, four times a day. By the age of 50, maximum frequency was 14 times a week, and by age 55 it was 8 times a week – a fairly sudden decline, but still a lot of sex.

Sexologists usually say you should have sex as often as it suits you. If you want to have sex twice a week, then have sex twice a week. If you want to have sex once a week, then have sex once a week. It's seems hard to argue with that. But I'm going to.

What does it really mean to 'want' sex? Very often it means waiting until your sex drive has built up sufficiently to overcome any 'negative' feelings – any inhibitions, for example, and, in particular, any resentments you might harbour towards your partner.

Some people are particularly good at being resentful. And this is the crazy thing; although a common reason for feeling resentful is not having enough sex, they actually react by withholding sex to 'punish' their partners. They then become all the more resentful as a result. It's bonkers but it happens.

These are the sort of thoughts that power the crisis along:

▶ *My partner doesn't deserve me.*
▶ *My partner doesn't deserve sex with me.*
▶ *My partner needs to be punished by my withholding sex.*

Recognize these thoughts? By thinking in this way, some people actually feed their own resentment. Every day without sex provides them with another justification for their negative feelings towards their partners. Then, finally, they can't stand not to have sex any longer. Their overpowering sex drives finally sweep all other considerations away and, afterwards, they feel contented.
For a while...

This can all sometimes make for explosive sexual encounters but it doesn't make for a great sex *life* nor for a great relationship. The way out of these destructive downward spirals is not to wait until you 'want' sex, but to have sex as a rhythmical part of your life.

You don't hold your breath until you're gasping for air, you don't wait to drink until you're dehydrated, and you don't put off eating until you're literally starving. So why not adopt the same attitude with sex? Why not treat it as something that you quite naturally and regularly do, without having to be 'desperate' for it?

Insight

When you choose to have sex before you're driven to it by – let's call it – lust, that's the creative act of *making* love. The other way is merely a discharge of sexual tension.

Between 1994 and 2000, another famous sex researcher, Shere Hite, asked women in the UK how often they desired sex. If you're a woman, you should already have a good idea of the answer. If you're a man you might be in for a surprise. Twenty-nine per cent of the women she interviewed said they wanted it daily, while a further 19 per cent wanted it 'a few times a week'. In other words, almost half of women desired sex several times a week, including the 29 per cent who wanted it every day.

Consequently, it probably isn't true to say that men want sex more often than women. In fact, older men are restrained by an ever-lengthening refractory period – the recovery time necessary before they can ejaculate again – and eventually, this can run into days. In Chapter 8, I explain how these men can keep up with their women by using the technique of multiple male orgasms.

Be a sex war pacifist

We all talk about the war of the sexes, and there's no doubt that, as far as a lot of people are concerned, there actually is one. Well, it may exist in the boardroom but don't let it enter your bedroom. Or your relationship.

Unfortunately, many men and women who say they're in love still compete with one another. They literally fight for superiority and dominance in the relationship. They take every opportunity to underline their partner's mistakes, including anything that goes wrong with sex. Eventually, one or both end up destroyed.

Ask yourself what sort of person you want as a partner. Someone whose confidence has been wrecked or someone who is self-assured, positive and optimistic? A partner with low self-esteem is a high price to pay to bolster your own sense of self-worth.

Lots of surveys show that the majority of women are dissatisfied with their partners when it comes to sex. In fact, far more women complain about their men than men complain about their women. It all comes down to the basic psychology of sex, which is that women have things done to them while men are responsible for the doing.

From this it follows that if women aren't having a great time, it must be the men's *fault*. (That's certainly how many men feel.) Yet men don't want to be bad lovers. Hopefully, your man cares enough about you to want to give you pleasure. So, if your man really isn't a great lover, it's probably out of ignorance rather than indifference. He may well imagine he's doing rather well, and if he doesn't know about your clitoris and all the other erogenous bits, well, there are plenty of women who don't know about them either. Don't be too hard on him; it's your job to explain to him what he's doing wrong and how he can improve.

Of course, there are also men who complain that their partners are unexciting. But women are not bad lovers on purpose any more than men are. Equally, if your wife or girlfriend doesn't know your penis needs lubricating or how much pressure to use on it, it's your job to explain.

WHEN WE'RE YOUNG WE'RE ALL BAD LOVERS

When we're young, we don't even know what we like ourselves or how to make ourselves happy, so we can hardly understand somebody else. Given luck we learn and things improve. If not, relationships break down.

In reality, there's no need for a sex war any more than there's a need for any war. Politicians still haven't learned how to solve world conflicts but, fortunately, you can put an end to conflict in your own relationship. Accept that men do not as a group deliberately set out to exploit or subjugate women and that women as a group do not deliberately set out to control or 'castrate' men. Don't knock your partner down. Build your partner up.

There was a man who hired a private detective because he thought his wife was having an affair. The detective followed the wife for a few days, then came back with his report. Yes, she'd been with another man. They'd been to the beach together, been boating together, been diving together, been to some nice restaurants, been dancing and, yes, there had been long and noisy sex. The husband looked ashen. 'Guess you never thought your wife would really have an affair,' said the detective. 'No, no, it's not that,' said the husband. 'I just never realized she could be so exciting.'

Be balanced

Only a very few things are important in life:

▶ *Your relationship with your partner is one of the most important things in your life.*
▶ *Sex is one of the most important things in your relationship.*
▶ *Who left the top off the toothpaste isn't important at all.*

10 THINGS TO REMEMBER

1 *The right mental attitude is as essential for great sex as any physical technique.*

2 *Being in love doesn't guarantee great sex, but you're even less likely to experience great sex if you're not in love.*

3 *If you've been brought up with negative feelings about sex, it's going to take time to become uninhibited, but it's essential that you do.*

4 *If you seem to be sexually incompatible don't despair because you may be able to become more compatible through communication.*

5 *Good communication equals good sex; bad communication equals bad sex.*

6 *The fundamental rule of good communication is that you don't criticize failure, you praise success.*

7 *Try not to turn down your partner's overtures.*

8 *Don't wait until you're 'desperate' for sex; this just creates tension and resentment in the relationship.*

9 *Don't let the 'sex war' enter your relationship or your bedroom.*

10 *Remember that your relationship is one of the most important things in your life, and that sex is one of the most important things in your relationship.*

HOW GREAT IS SEX NOW?

▶ *Have you made progress in tackling your inhibitions?*   Yes/No

▶ *Are you sleeping naked together?*   Yes/No

▶ *Have you told your partner something new about your sexual desires?*   Yes/No

▶ *Are you showing your partner more affection than you give your pet?*   Yes/No

▶ *Are you doing something sexual together (not necessarily intercourse) most days?*   Yes/No

▶ *If you're a woman, have you taken control of sex on at least one occasion this week?*   Yes/No

▶ *If you're a man, have you let your partner take control of sex on at least one occasion this week?*   Yes/No

If you answered 'no' to more than two questions, re-read the relevant parts of the chapter and make an effort to put the suggestions into effect. This is all about breaking down your inhibitions and learning to express yourself sexually. A good test is: are you able to tell your partner *all* the things you'd like to do and *all* the things you'd like done, without embarrassment? Remember that the happier your sex life with your partner, the happier all of your life will be.

2

....

Women's bodies

In this chapter you will learn:
- *how your body works sexually (if you're a woman)*
- *how your partner's body works sexually (if you're a man)*
- *how to use your knowledge for great sex.*

In this chapter we're going to take a look at women's bodies.
If you're a woman, you need to understand how your own body
works if you're going to both give and receive the maximum
pleasure. If you're a man, you need to understand your partner's
body so that you know how to give pleasure and how to take it.

A woman's body is an incredible thing (and so is a man's, but
we come to that in Chapter 3). The more you discover about it,
the more fantastic you realize it is. It's composed of something
like 10,000 trillion cells. I have to say 'something like' because,
understandably, it's not all that easy to count them. Every one
of those cells is a universe on its own, containing some 20,000
different types of protein, totalling maybe 100 million protein
molecules. That's, well, an awful lot of molecules.

I'm telling you this for two reasons. First, I just want you to
appreciate how complicated the body is and the importance of
looking after it. Second, I want you to understand the scale of
the problem in unravelling how a woman's body works sexually.
If you are a woman, then, fortunately, you have a simple and

traditional alternative to electron microscopes and piles of medical encyclopaedias. To understand your own sexual response you only have to masturbate.

Great masturbation

More than half a century ago, 62 per cent of women interviewed by the pioneering sex researcher Alfred Kinsey admitted to masturbation. A quarter of a century later, the feminist sex researcher Shere Hite put the figure at 82 per cent and, today, it's almost certainly higher. Some women masturbate on a daily basis, some once or twice a week, some once a month, but the vast majority of women do it, irrespective of age. Women are just as likely to masturbate when in a relationship as when they're not. Masturbation, after all, is different to sex with a partner.

Now that's cleared up, we can discuss the subject openly. There's absolutely no need to feel guilty about it. If you do, try reading Chapter 1 again. In fact, you'd have to be crazy *not* to masturbate, given the pleasure it creates and the huge number of benefits, some of which are listed below.

If you're a woman who, until now, hasn't experienced orgasm from intercourse, get masturbating right away. If you don't orgasm easily even from masturbation, it may be that you're just not putting enough into it.

....

Insight

It's significant that women who don't masturbate are far more likely to be women who don't orgasm during sex with a partner. To help you feel more relaxed about the whole thing, it's worth reflecting on the lengths some women go to – ice cubes in the vagina, dressing up, acting out fantasies, and much more. If you want to confirm that or get inspiration have a look at 'Taking it further'. It's also a good idea to

(Contd)

examine yourself in a mirror and get comfortable with the way you are. Take my word for it – whatever you may think of your genitals, men will love them and so should you.

Shere Hite (*The New Hite Report*, 1976, is recommended reading for everybody) classified techniques for masturbation into seven main categories and numerous sub-types. If you've only been trying one way, then try some others. The main classifications are using your hand on your clitoral/vulval area while lying on your back, or alternatively while lying on your stomach, thrusting against an object, pressing thighs together rhythmically, using a jet of water, inserting something into the vagina and, finally, any other technique. Some women say they can only orgasm with their legs open, while others can only orgasm with their legs together. Try both.

Insight

I suspect that at least some of the women who say they can't orgasm with their legs open simply aren't opening them far enough. The key is to create tension and if you're a woman who doesn't orgasm easily you'll need to maximize it by opening your legs as far as physically possible. Lifting them up in the air will increase tension even further.

11 REASONS WHY WOMEN SHOULD MASTURBATE

1 *Masturbation teaches you how to orgasm.*
2 *Masturbation relieves tension.*
3 *Masturbation helps to develop your sexual responsiveness.*
4 *Masturbation teaches you about your own body.*
5 *Masturbation helps you learn techniques in private before trying with a partner.*
6 *Masturbation helps you to understand your partner's body.*
7 *Masturbation provides the sexual activity vital to mental and physical health when no partner is available.*
8 *Masturbation makes you happy.*
9 *Masturbation is readily available.*
10 *Masturbation is free.*
11 *Masturbation is safe.*

Most women say that the orgasms they have during masturbation are more intense than those from intercourse. In fact, the famous sex scientists William Masters and Virginia Johnson found that women's orgasms from masturbation produced higher heart rates than for any other type of orgasm, female or male. Nevertheless, most women also say that orgasms from intercourse affect more of their bodies and that they prefer them to masturbatory orgasms.

Why should there be this difference? There seem to be several reasons. First, during masturbation, you receive bio-feedback that allows you to act with complete precision. A partner, being unable to receive that bio-feedback, cannot perform with the same accuracy (although good communication can help). Second, you may feel less inhibited on your own. Third, the uterus may have something to do with it (see page 30). Fourth, during intercourse the vagina is certainly restricted by the presence of the penis (and, equally, the penis is restricted by the vagina).

Yet masturbation isn't only about relief and pleasure. In the film *Love And Death*, a woman tells Woody Allen's character that he's the greatest lover she's ever known. To which he replies: 'Well, I practise a lot when I'm on my own.' A funny line and also true. Masturbation is a way of practising so that you'll know what you've got to do to feel good and what your partner's got to do. Don't forget to tell him. Masturbation can also help you to understand your *partner's* body to a degree. The fact is that women's and men's bodies are far more alike than most people realize, as you'll see in the next chapter. So, take plenty of time to explore. Try different techniques to see what works and what doesn't. Try stimulating different places. If a place you know is erogenous in others doesn't work for you, then spend some time on it regularly. The aim is to awaken the sensuality of as many parts of your body as possible.

Insight

For great sex, you're sometimes going to need to play with your clitoris during intercourse. Get comfortable with the

(Contd)

idea of letting your partner see you masturbate. Guys, don't be offended, it's no reflection on your skills. If your partner feels free to masturbate during sex with you, she's going to appreciate sex with you even more.

Women's 'bits'

This section details all of a woman's important 'bits', but excluding the mind, which is dealt with in Chapter 7.

THE CLITORIS

The clitoris is the principal source of pleasure in both masturbation and intercourse. It's often said that it's a recent discovery, but you only have to read old erotic texts or look at old erotic paintings and prints to know that isn't true. However, it is true that the existence of the clitoris wasn't common knowledge in the West even a mere 50 years ago. Nowadays, that seems almost unbelievable, given the easy and intense pleasure it's capable of creating.

In most women, the clitoral glans (the really sensitive bit) is around the size of a lentil (but some are much larger) and it nestles under a 'hood' above the entrance to the vagina where the inner lips meet. Above the hood is the 'shaft'. The hood and the shaft are the visible parts and are what most people refer to as 'the clitoris' although, as we'll see in a moment, there's much more.

The distance between the clitoris and the vagina varies from woman to woman but a penis shuttling backwards and forwards in the vagina will never provide the clitoris with much direct stimulation. That stimulation *must* be provided in other ways. When excited, the clitoris enlarges and hardens a little and, later, actually retracts. At that stage, you (or your partner) might not be able to find it.

What many people still don't realize even today is that the visible
clitoris is only the tip of a much larger structure known as the
'clitoral system', which is hidden inside and is analogous to the
penis. Just as the penis has two 'tubes' that fill with blood to
cause erection, so women have two 'tubes' either side of the outer
third of the vagina, which also fill with blood. Women also have
a sizeable erection but, apart from the vaginal lips, it can't really
be seen.

Facts about the clitoris

▶ *The clitoris contains 8,000 nerve fibres, twice as many as the
penis.*

▶ *The clitoris enlarges with excitement and becomes more rigid.*

▶ *The clitoris retracts once a woman becomes very excited.*

▶ *The clitoris that you can see and touch is only the tip of a
clitoral system that comprises 18 different parts.*

> **Have a go**
>
> You probably already use your clitoris to masturbate and are
> very familiar with it. But possibly you're not aware that the
> hood can be retracted by gently pulling back on the shaft or
> by pulling the skin of your pubic mound up towards your
> navel. That will then expose the tiny, bright red glans, which
> is the most sensitive part. Try to work out exactly what feels
> good so you can tell your partner precisely where and how to
> stimulate you and with what rhythm.

Tips for men

The clitoris is analogous to the penis and, equally, needs to be treated with different amounts of pressure at different times. Also bear in mind that no two women are exactly the same. Most women prefer stimulation to begin a little above the clitoris (on the hood or shaft) or to the side or, if they're very sensitive, even through their underwear. Later, you can tantalize the glans itself with flicks of your tongue. To expose the glans you'll need to retract the hood by very, very gently spreading the labia (see 'The vulva', page 31) or by pushing the skin on the pubic mound up towards the navel.

After orgasm the clitoris – rather like the glans of the penis – may be too delicate to be touched for a few seconds. Where women differ from men is that when they have sexy thoughts or see or hear something stimulating, they're not generally aware of any erection of the clitoris. The response of which they are aware, as you'll see in the next section, is lubrication of the vagina.

THE VAGINA

The vagina is the place where a man has to put his penis if reproduction is to take place and yet, pleasurable as it is for the man, the vagina is not the main instrument of pleasure for a woman. Only around a third of women can orgasm from intercourse alone. That's the first mystery, for surely evolution should have favoured a pleasure-sensitive vagina? In fact, only the outer third of the vagina, amounting to an inch or so, is very sensitive at all, partly because there are more nerve endings there and partly because the entrance is surrounded by the clitoral system. The proof of this is that very few women masturbate by inserting anything into their vaginas.

Before we examine the issue of clitoral versus vaginal orgasms any further, let's take a look deeper inside. Beyond the entrance, on the roof of the vagina, lies the renowned G-spot. The G-spot is so important that it gets its very own entry (see page 27). The cervix is the little rubbery bit that protrudes at the far end of the vagina and is the entrance to the uterus or womb. It's shaped like the end of a broom handle and is quite pliable. The ovaries lie on either side, beyond the end of the vagina.

When a woman feels sexy, the walls of the vagina 'sweat' beads of lubricant. In a young woman, the 'sweating' begins within 10–30 seconds (longer in an older woman), and she'll be well aware of it. In that sense, lubrication is equivalent to erection of the penis as a sort of bio-feedback of arousal. Once a high level of sexual excitement has been reached, lubrication actually reduces in all women. So when lovemaking is extended, be sure to use some additional lubrication. The wall of the vagina also swells as excitement builds.

This brings us to the second mystery. For those women who *do* orgasm from intercourse alone, *how* does it happen? Despite decades of quite meticulous research, the issue is still controversial. It's only in certain positions that the clitoris receives any direct stimulation at all from a man's thrusting. Some experts argue that it's the indirect stimulating of the clitoris that does it, the sort of pulling of the surrounding tissues as the penis moves in and out. Others argue that bumping against the cervix at the far end of the vagina has something to do with it. Still others point to the G-spot.

Insight

My own opinion is that it's never possible to stimulate the vagina *alone*, because, at the very least, the mind will also be stimulated, and that, as you shall see in Chapter 7, is extremely powerful.

What does seem to have been established almost beyond doubt by William Masters and Virginia Johnson is that, no matter what the source of stimulation that causes an orgasm, the vaginal response patterns are always the same. In other words, it doesn't make any difference to the vagina if orgasm is achieved by intercourse, stimulation of the clitoris, stimulation of the mons area (the little mound covered by the triangle of pubic hair), stimulation of the nipples or, even, by simply fantasizing about sex.

Yet many women insist that clitorally-induced orgasms are quite different to those produced by intercourse. They say that orgasms from clitoral stimulation are more localized, whereas those from intercourse are more profound and affect more of the body. So what's going on? The answer may not be in the vagina but in the uterus (see page 30).

Facts about the vagina

▶ *The vagina is surprisingly small, measuring just 2 cm (0.8 inches) in diameter and approximately 7.5 cm (3 inches) in length (in women who haven't had children).*

▶ *The vagina enlarges during sexual excitement, ballooning to around 6 cm (2.3 inches) diameter at the cervix end and lengthening to around 10 cm (4 inches).*

▶ *The vagina stretches to accommodate the penis, whatever its size.*

▶ *During orgasm the outer third of the vagina contracts at intervals of 0.8 seconds. Most women experience three to five contractions, but there could be as many as 10 to 15.*

Have a go

Explore your vagina with your fingers. Find out which parts feel responsive and which parts produce no sensation at all. If you have fairly long fingers, you should be able to touch your cervix. You'll also want to pay particular attention to the G-spot area (see following page).

Tips for men
The vagina, as you saw above, is actually very small (so there's
no need for you to worry about *your* size). Do not just push in
and begin thrusting away. That could cause pain, not pleasure,
especially if you bump against an ovary. Allow time for the vagina
to stretch to your size.

THE G-SPOT AREA AND FEMALE EJACULATION

Does the G-spot really exist? Does female ejaculation really exist?
These are the questions people so often ask in my focus groups.
And the answers are that, yes, the G-spot *does* exist and that, yes,
many women do spurt from the urethra after their G-spots have
been stimulated. But, if this is so, why doesn't everybody know
about it? One man I interviewed had had sex with 400 women and
yet hadn't ever observed it. The answer is that the liquid exists, but
usually the quantity is so small as to be almost invisible. The only
controversy is over what exactly is the liquid.

The G-spot is named after the German researcher Ernst
Gräfenberg, although he himself never referred to it as a 'spot'.
It's actually about the size of a thumbnail and some sexologists
call it the 'G-spot area'. It's the part of the vagina behind which
lies the female prostate, sometimes referred to as 'Skene's glands'.
When you rub or press this area, you stimulate the female prostate
through the wall of the vagina. It produces a fluid comparable to
the male prostatic fluid (a major constituent of semen), which is
expelled into the urethra, the tube through which women urinate.
The urethra, of course, has its outlet just above the entrance to the
vagina and just below the clitoris. A small quantity of liquid would
be almost indistinguishable from lubricant coming from the vagina.
But some women, as you'll see, claim to ejaculate large quantities
of fluid, up to a cupful and sometimes even more.

The G-spot area is on the roof of the vagina, and in the majority of
women it's actually just inside the entrance. After pushing a finger

through the resistance of the opening, the G-spot is the very next thing your finger will encounter on the roof. You'll know it at once because it'll feel slightly corrugated. This 'roughness' increases with sexual excitement so, if you can't find it, wait until things have hotted up a bit. Go beyond the spot and the vagina will feel incredibly smooth. And that's all there is to it. Smooth means too far, rough is right. (However, in a proportion of women, maybe a quarter to a third, the G-spot is further back.)

The women who are most enthusiastic about the G-spot area are also those who claim to ejaculate large quantities of liquid. They soak the bed. They say female ejaculation takes sex to new heights both for them and for their partners. They say the physical sensations are intense and the emotional sensations even stronger. Yet given the small size of the female prostate, how can such large quantities of liquid be possible?

Devotees of female ejaculation insist it isn't urine, but my opinion is that when there's a large quantity of liquid it is mostly urine, slightly altered by the release of hormones during sex, and with the addition of prostatic fluid from the female prostate. My guess is that, somehow, massaging the G-spot area releases the bladder sphincter, which would normally be shut during sex, and thus urine is let out. When this happens during orgasm, the contractions of the vagina and uterus squeeze the bladder and, if it's full, the urine actually squirts out under pressure. (And, in fact, the bladder quite often does fill up more rapidly during sex.)

Insight

In the end, it doesn't really matter where the fluid comes from. It's just a question of what you (and your partner) enjoy. If you like it, do it. If you don't, don't.

Learning to ejaculate

If you've never ejaculated but think you'd like to try, the best way to acquire the ability is alone and in the bath. There are two stages. The first is to learn to orgasm and urinate simultaneously. The second is to convert what you've learned into 'proper' ejaculation.

For stage one, first drink a couple of glasses of water and wait until your bladder feels a little full. Then get into the bath, naked, and begin to masturbate. Once things are coming along nicely, slip a couple of fingers or a dildo inside and apply pressure to your G-spot. If you can't find it, re-read the section above. With your other hand, continue working on your clitoris. The aim is to co-ordinate your orgasm with an overwhelming need to urinate. When your bladder feels as if it will burst and you think you can hold back neither orgasm nor urination, press out and relax your pelvic muscles.

Insight

Psychologically it isn't easy to 'let go', which is the reason for sitting in the bath where there's no problem about making a mess. Some women find it helps to shout out loud: 'Yes! Yes! Yes!' or something similar. The more force behind the urination the more pleasure.

Once you're adept at ejaculating urine you can experiment without drinking beforehand. Since you won't have a full bladder it won't be quite as easy. You'll know you're close to the point when the G-spot area is hard to the touch, it feels as if you need to urinate, and you also feel close to orgasm. Build the sensations to a peak by pushing repeatedly for a few moments, as if you were urinating, while keeping the finger on your G-spot still. Then remove your finger from your vagina and push again, exactly as if you were pushing to urinate. This time, since your bladder is fairly empty, any liquid should come from your prostate not your bladder, and it should give you a new sensation.

Insight

If you find you can ejaculate from your prostate, and it gives you an extra thrill, all well and good. If not, you may nevertheless still wish to ejaculate from your bladder, if you find it exciting. Some women find they can squirt a little urine with each orgasm. Discuss it with your partner. Some men may not like it but others will be very excited to be part of such a special experience. You'll probably want to protect the bed with a couple of towels.

Tips for men

Have a go at locating your partner's G-spot, as described above. In Chapters 5 and 6 you're going to be stimulating it with your fingers and your penis. If it works, you're going to be getting wet, so get used to the idea.

THE UTERUS

Not many men or even women understand the significance of the uterus (or womb) when it comes to sex, but it's capable of a powerful and highly pleasurable orgasm.

Given that the uterus can contain a baby, it's actually amazingly small when not in use. It's the shape of a pear (the widest part at the top) and measures just 7.5 cm (3 inches) long and 5 cm (2 inches) wide (in a woman who's never been pregnant).

When a woman becomes sexually excited, the uterus responds by tilting back from its usual position and rising up. It may also increase significantly in size (this is more pronounced in women who've given birth).

Just how the uterus does orgasm is, like so much to do with sex, the subject of controversy. Some sexologists argue that the uterus only contracts as a result of particularly successful vaginal stimulation. (Uterine muscles also contract during labour, which is one of the reasons some women are advised to avoid sex in the weeks immediately prior to their due date.) This, if true, would explain why women register orgasm from intercourse as something more 'profound'. But William Masters and Virginia Johnson frequently observed uterine contractions from clitoral masturbation, and said the contractions were more intense than those from intercourse although not necessarily as satisfying.

What's certain is that the contractions start within two to four seconds of a woman feeling that orgasm has begun, and at the usual 0.8 second intervals. They are powerful enough to expel menstrual fluid right out of the vagina during a woman's period.

> **Have a go**
> When you have orgasms, see if you can work out whether or not they involve the uterus and, if so, what was the cause.

Tips for men
Uterine orgasm seems to require a high degree of vasocongestion (blood rushing to the area), so take your time.

THE VULVA

Most of what a man sees when a woman opens her legs is covered by the word 'vulva'. This includes the clitoris, of course, which was dealt with above. Nothing else is as sensitive but, even so, it all produces extremely pleasant feelings. The 'mons' is the little mound covered in hair. The opening of the vagina is also included as part of the vulva. Either side are the 'labia majora', the outer lips, and the 'labia minora', the inner lips. The labia majora are hair-covered and not particularly sensitive, because their job is to protect. When a woman is excited, they pull back to reveal the labia minora, although in a woman who has had children this may not be so clear. In most women the labia minora are incredibly smooth but there's nothing abnormal about inner labia that are textured. As they enlarge with excitement, the labia minora effectively increase the length of the vagina by around 1 cm (1/2 inch). They also become significant sources of pleasure when stimulated by fingers or the penis. Just above the vaginal opening, the urethral opening is so tiny as to be invisible, but stimulation of the G-spot can cause it to widen. Some women find the urethral opening a source of extra pleasure but most don't.

> **Have a go**
> Be positive about your vulva and get used to the idea of displaying it to your lover. If you haven't used a mirror to become familiar with it then do so now. And if you're not used to thinking of your vulva as beautiful then get that idea
> *(Contd)*

Tips for men
The colour change in the labia minora is a sure sign of how well
you're doing. If the inner labia have gone from pink to bright red
then, provided you continue, your partner is certain to orgasm.

THE BREASTS AND NIPPLES

Sensitivity of the breasts and nipples to stimulation varies
enormously from woman to woman. Some feel very little, some
find it highly pleasurable, and some can actually orgasm this way.
How many? That's difficult to say because it all depends on the
stimulation. A man in one of my focus groups told me he had
brought women to orgasm by caressing their breasts even though
the women themselves didn't consider their breasts to be especially
sensitive. He also told me that it took about one hour.

Facts about breasts and nipples
- *There's no connection between breast size and sensitivity.*
- *Excitement can increase the length of nipples by as much as
  1 cm (0.4 inches).*
- *Excitement can increase breast size by as much as 25 per cent
  (less for older women and those who have breast-fed their
  children).*
- *Excitement can cause a pink mottling of the breasts as well as
  increased visibility of the veins.*
- *One breast may be more sensitive than the other.*

Have a go
When masturbating, play with your breasts to see what kind
of stimulation works. Does stroking the skin do anything?
Tickling the nipples? Rolling them between your fingers?
How much pressure is good?

Tips for men
Erection of the nipples is the first visible sign that a woman is
sexually excited. Most women like attention to their breasts but
don't forget that they can be particularly tender just before a
period.

THE ANUS AND RECTUM

You may think of your anus as something of a no-go area but, in
fact, it's absolutely packed with nerve endings and, what's more,
its contractions are part of your orgasm (but over the age of 50 or
so it usually stops contracting). So you should really learn to love
it and use it as part of your sex play. It's not 'dirty' but a part of
your body that's capable of producing some interesting effects.
If you never have any kind of anal stimulation you're missing out
on a whole dimension.

Facts about the anus and rectum
▶ *The anus is opened and closed by a ring of muscle governed*
   by the central nervous system and is therefore under conscious
   control.
▶ *Inside the anus is the anal canal, which measures between*
   2.5 cm and 5 cm (1–2 inches).
▶ *The anal canal is capable of generating highly pleasurable*
   sensations and never contains waste matter.
▶ *At the inside end of the anal canal, the interior sphincter*
   is governed by the autonomic nervous system and is not
   therefore under conscious control.
▶ *Beyond the interior sphincter is the rectum, which is free of*
   waste matter for significant periods.
▶ *Unlike the vagina, the anal canal and rectum produce no*
   lubrication so artificial lubrication is absolutely essential
   (see Chapter 9).

There are effectively three levels of anal play. The first is external,
that's to say, simply rubbing the outside with a lubricated finger.
The second is slipping a lubricated fingertip (nail well trimmed)

inside, into the anal canal (a technique known as *postillionage*). The third is penetration of your anus and rectum by a 'butt plug', vibrator, or your partner's penis.

If you've not yet experienced any kind of anal stimulation at all you may be feeling somewhat mystified, to say the least. To which I can only say, try it. The surprising consensus among women who do it is that the anus is more or less on a par with the vagina in terms of sensitivity. However, it's what might be called a 'sympathetic area'. It only gets excited when your clitoris is excited and rarely gets excited all on its own. So touching your anus before you feel hot probably won't do anything for you at all. But once you're really motoring and blood has rushed to the area, the effect can be electric. And that 'sympathy' works both ways. As your anal area becomes increasingly sensitized, so it intensifies sensations in your genitals. What's more, anal play isn't solely about physical pleasure, it's also about psychology. It feels like the ultimate act of offering yourself. That may be of limited significance when you're on your own, but when you're with a partner you love and trust it can be an incredibly powerful experience. In her book *The Surrender*, Toni Bentley has even called it an experience of God.

Insight

You might have certain fears about anal play, which I'll deal with here. First of all, if your finger or toy goes no further than the anal canal there can't possibly be any mess at all. If you want deeper penetration (which might be the case with a partner) then it's all a matter of timing, as I'll be explaining in Chapter 5. As regards physical damage, no harm can result from the *gentle* penetration of the anus or internal sphincter by a finger (with closely trimmed nail), properly designed sex toy or penis, *provided plenty of artificial lubricant is used*. The muscles will not be weakened nor left gaping open.

The transmission of infections, however, is quite a different matter. Obviously, nothing that has been in the anal canal or rectum should subsequently be used on the vulva or in the vagina unless it has been scrupulously washed. Never have anal sex with a man unless you're 100 per cent positive he's free of diseases that could be transmitted to you. So this isn't something for casual lovers, only committed long-term partners. Psychologically, too, anal sex is all about complete trust, not quick thrills.

Have a go

Once you're already excited, explore your anal area with a lubricated finger. Try running it round and round the rim. Try backwards and forwards. If that feels nice, insert your finger into your anus as far as the first finger joint, while you continue masturbating. You should immediately notice an intensification of sexual feelings and may have an orgasm as a result. That may be as far as you want to go at first and there's certainly no need to rush. But once you've become relaxed about the whole idea of anal stimulation you may want to take it a bit further than just a fingertip. Stretching the opening with two, three or even four fingers will have an even more powerful effect. If you opt for a vibrator, be sure it's of a design that can't possibly disappear inside – the muscles can exert an unbelievable 'suction'. (See Chapter 9 for more advice on anal sex toys).

As regards anal sex with a partner, I'm sure you can remember the first time you ever had intercourse and it probably wasn't great. Nevertheless you continued to have sex because you believed things would get a lot better. Well, the first time you have anal sex probably won't be great either. So don't take that as proof it can never be any good. Just as intercourse gets better and better, so can anal sex. However, it's more tricky and calls for a partner who is both considerate and skilful. Getting used to playing with your own anus before you ever try anything with a man will make things go a lot better. I'll have more to say about anal sex with a partner in Chapter 5.

Tips for men

Anal sex is a subject that nowadays causes a lot of rows. Don't make a big issue out of it or try to rush things if you're partner isn't ready. A little stimulation of her anal area during cunnilingus might be a beginning. If she's happy with that you might move on to slipping a lubricated fingertip into her anus when intercourse is approaching a climax – easiest when she's on top or in the 'Cuddly Bears' position (see Chapter 6). It's a good idea to make one hand your 'anal hand' and the other your 'vaginal hand' so you don't get mixed up about which finger went where – nothing that has been in her anus or rectum should ever be used on her vulva or vagina until it's been washed. As regards full anal sex, it takes a lot of patience and skill (and masses of lubrication) to be pleasurable for her. Badly done, it can hurt a lot. I'll be explaining all about the right way in Chapter 5.

THE PERINEAL SPONGE

Behind the perineum, the small area between the anus and the vagina, there's erectile tissue known as the 'perineal sponge'. It lines the front floor of the vagina and, when stimulated, it can feel very pleasant. Stimulation can be achieved by stroking the perineum or, more successfully, via the vagina or anus or, in a technique to be discussed in Chapter 5, by both simultaneously.

Have a go

Try stimulating your perineum and see what happens. Try featherlight touches, firmer caresses and rubbing. Now try to stimulate the perineal sponge through the floor of the vagina or, alternatively, via the anus.

Tips for men

The perineum is unlikely to produce any fireworks, but it can provide an additional source of mild pleasure, just as your own does to you.

THE HEAD

Eyes
The eyes are one of the major organs of arousal. Through them a woman sees the soft lighting, the candles, her own body, her partner's body, her partner's excitement and all the rest. In them, her partner sees her response.

Ears
The ears can be nibbled, sucked and blown into. Incidentally, a woman's ears have one other function. They're also for hearing the romantic and exciting things a man should be saying, and for listening to music.

Nose
The nose responds not only to nice perfumes but also to male pheromones. In fact, in my focus groups, a man's smell turned out to be the most consistently significant aphrodisiac for women.

Hair
The hair is a turn-on for a man, and, for a woman it feels tingly when a man runs his hands through it.

Neck
The neck is probably the best place for a man to start arousing his partner physically (after, that is, arousing her mentally). The back of the neck is particularly effective. There's almost certainly a link there with the mating behaviour of many animals, in which the male bites the female's neck.

Tongue
Most women love kissing far more than men do. Sucking and biting (gently) the tongue can be very exciting because the tongue is connected to the same set of nerves as the genitals.

Have a go
Check your response to pictures of naked men, to different kinds of music and to various aromas.

Tips for men
Be willing to pay a lot of attention, in various different ways, to your partner's head.

THE SKIN

The skin is actually the body's largest organ. We've already looked at some very particular areas of skin, but women can enjoy being touched just about anywhere, as long as it's done in the right way. The sex flush that begins on the breasts can, with intense excitement, also spread across the skin of the abdomen and shoulders and, when orgasm is close, even across the thighs, buttocks and back.

Have a go
When masturbating, tickle your skin all over. Where feels best (apart, of course, from the genitals)?

Tips for men
Take your time, because the sensitivity of the skin increases slowly. Try the toes and the backs of the knees.

THE PC MUSCLE

A woman's internal sexual apparatus is supported by a group of muscles known as the pubococcygeus muscles, pelvic floor muscles, or more popularly as the 'PC muscle'. The stronger it is, the more powerful your orgasms will be. What's more, by flexing your PC muscle, you can actually stroke your partner's penis inside your vagina. A toned PC muscle is one of the keys to great sex.

Exactly where is the PC muscle? It runs from the pubic bone to the base of the spine, and it's the same muscle you use to hold back when you feel the need to urinate. If you're not sure which muscle it is, try stopping the flow of urine next time you go to the toilet. That's the muscle. If you can't stop the flow of urine, the muscle is definitely weak.

You can exercise your PC simply by contracting it. You can do it quite invisibly while driving a car, sitting at a desk or watching television. Start with, say, ten contractions repeated three times over and build up from there. A full exercise programme for the PC muscle is given in Chapter 11.

> ### Have a go
> Do the PC exercises regularly.

Tips for men
Encourage your partner to do her PC exercises by doing your own (see Chapter 3).

TEN THINGS EVERY MAN SHOULD KNOW ABOUT WOMEN

1 *Only a small minority of women orgasm as a result of intercourse alone.*
2 *Women orgasm primarily by stimulation of the clitoris.*
3 *The thrusting of intercourse only provides minimal stimulation of the clitoris.*
4 *If you don't stimulate her clitoris with your tongue or fingers, she'll have to do it herself.*
5 *Ideally, a woman wants several orgasms before you have yours.*
6 *After the first orgasm, subsequent orgasms usually come more easily.*
7 *Many women say their final orgasm is much stronger than the preceding ones if timed with their partner's ejaculation.*
8 *Women take much longer to come down from their sexual high than men do, which is why the period afterwards is so important.*
9 *Women have more erogenous zones than men and they like them to be used.*
10 *The vagina needs to be lubricated by sexual excitement or artificial lubricant before you enter; the anus always needs artificial lubricant.*

What happens during sex?

Now we know about all the bits, we can try to understand what actually happens during sex. From there, we can start to work out how we can enhance sexual pleasure. The whole sexual experience can be divided into four phases:

1 *Excitement phase (when sexual tension builds rapidly)*
2 *Plateau phase (in which the tension is maintained or continues to grow slowly)*
3 *Orgasm (which releases the tension)*
4 *Resolution phase (in which things gradually return to normal).*

Of course, many women can experience the plateau and orgasm phases several times during a single lovemaking session.

During sexual excitement, two particular things happen:

▶ *vasocongestion*
▶ *myotonia.*

These are the technical words used by sexologists to describe changes in the body with which we're all familiar. 'Vasocongestion' is simply the build-up of blood, especially in the pelvic organs. It also causes a 'sex flush' on the skin. The important thing to remember is that vasocongestion continues building up and building up, even over a period of hours.

'Myotonia' simply means increased muscular tension. This can happen all over the body and is why we all pull faces when excitement rises. It's partly involuntary and partly voluntary.

These reactions and lots of others (including breathing rate, heart rate and blood pressure) are controlled by a mass of chemicals, including adrenaline (epinephrine), noradrenaline (norepinephrine), dopamine, nitric oxide, opioids, oxytocin, phenylethylamine or PEA, and serotonin.

WHAT IS AN ORGASM?

Any woman who's ever had an orgasm knows what the feeling is like, but putting it into words is very difficult, as even poets have discovered. Scientists don't have that problem. They simply attach electrodes and insert cameras and, hey presto, very soon they can describe it ... in terms of quantities of PEA and dopamine, numbers of contractions per second and all the rest.

One way of explaining an orgasm is as a release of the tension that builds up in what we've called the excitement and plateau phases. It's rather like winding up an elastic band. The more you twist it, the more violently it unravels. In other words, the longer you make love (within reason) the more powerful the orgasm.

The key places for this tension to build and release include the PC muscle, which may contract approximately eight to 12 times, followed by the vaginal and uterine muscles.

Yet why does orgasm feel so nice? Because there's also a sort of 'orgasm' in the brain. Not a physical spasm in this case but a release of 'happy' chemicals. Let's take a closer look at some of the chemicals I mentioned earlier:

▶ *Dopamine gets into the frontal lobe of the brain during orgasm and produces a feeling of bliss. (Incidentally, it also dulls feelings of pain so you could try sex instead of an aspirin.)*
▶ *PEA peaks during orgasm – it is an amphetamine-like substance that makes you feel like you're walking on air. The more of this you have, the more you'll maintain (or get back) those euphoric feelings from the early days of your love affair. PEA combined with dopamine and the stress-reducing noradrenaline makes an even more potent combination. Incidentally, you can increase your noradrenaline level by ten times with just eight minutes of vigorous exercise.*
▶ *Oxytocin is a chemical that, among other things, sensitizes nerves and stimulates muscle contraction. It's also a very*

'romantic' hormone because it creates a sense of attachment to another person (and, incidentally, a mother's attachment to her new baby). The more oxytocin going around the more likely you and your partner will stay together.

▶ *Serotonin makes you feel content (which is why it's an ingredient in drugs to treat depression). It's all part of that satisfied feeling you have after sex and it also initiates sleep, which is one of the reasons why you might feel like a nap after orgasm.*

These are just four of the chemicals. You can see now why simultaneous orgasm is so special. If you don't orgasm together, one of you will be wanting to go to sleep while the other is still in a state of tension. If you do orgasm together, you'll both experience bliss. How this is achieved is explained in Chapter 6.

THE KEYS TO GREAT ORGASMS

The reason why I listed all those chemicals in the last section is the same reason why I've detailed what happens in the sex organs. I want you to understand that sex is a very complicated process that makes huge demands on the body and that, inevitably, takes time if the full response is to develop. Putting together everything we've learned we can see that:

▶ *If you're going to respond to the maximum during sex, you have to have a healthy body and a healthy diet (because those chemicals don't come out of nowhere).*
▶ *You have to allow plenty of time to give your body the opportunity to develop the maximum response.*
▶ *The more blood you can get into those key areas, the more sensitive you'll be.*
▶ *The more tension you can build up in those key muscles, and the stronger the muscles, the bigger the orgasm.*

We'll be looking at how to achieve all those things later on, but in the next chapter we take a look at men's bodies.

Periods and sexual desire

Most women say there's a time (or times) in their monthly cycle when they naturally feel more sexual desire. However, curiously, different women feel at their maximum at different stages of the cycle. Some women say this is about halfway through the cycle, that is, around the time of ovulation, whereas others say just before a period or during a period. In fact there's no *physiological* reason not to have intercourse or masturbate during menstruation. Some women find that orgasm actually relieves discomfort and speeds up the whole process of menstruation.

10 THINGS TO REMEMBER

1   Masturbation is a non-negotiable, essential part of your
    sex life.

2   The clitoris is just the tip of a much larger organ, the clitoral
    system, which is analogous to the penis.

3   Only around a third of women can orgasm from intercourse
    alone.

4   Clitoral orgasms are described as being more 'intense' than
    orgasms provoked in the vagina, but less 'satisfying'.

5   The G-spot does exist – it's the area of the vaginal wall behind
    which lies the female prostate.

6   Women can ejaculate.

7   The uterus (womb) has orgasms.

8   Other sexually important places include the vulva, breasts,
    anus, perineum, eyes and ears.

9   Orgasms can be intensified by strengthening the PC muscle
    and by creating maximum vasocongestion and muscle tension.

10 Artificial lubricants enhance pleasure and are essential for
    anal play.

HOW GREAT IS SEX NOW?

▶ *Are you masturbating more often and more happily?*   Yes/No

▶ *Have you found new ways of masturbating?*   Yes/No

▶ *Have you examined your genitals in a mirror?*   Yes/No

▶ *Have you found and stimulated your G-spot?*   Yes/No

▶ *Have you had a go at ejaculating?*   Yes/No

▶ *Have you discovered which of your breasts is the most sensitive?*   Yes/No

▶ *Have you explored anal sensation?*   Yes/No

▶ *Have you identified your PC muscle and flexed it?*   Yes/No

If you answered 'no' to more than three questions, re-read the relevant parts of the chapter and make an effort to put the suggestions into effect. Remember that women who masturbate frequently tend to be more orgasmic with their partners. You need to be comfortable with your own body before you can have great sex with another person. Don't feel guilty about masturbation. It's normal and it's good. So get exploring and enjoy yourself.

3

Men's bodies

In this chapter you will learn:
- *how your body works sexually (if you're a man)*
- *how your partner's body works sexually (if you're a woman)*
- *how to use your knowledge for great sex.*

In this chapter we're going to take a look at men's bodies. If you're a man, you need to understand how your own body works if you're going to both give and receive the maximum pleasure. If you're a woman, you need to understand your partner's body so that you know how to give pleasure and how to take it.

According to the Bible, God created men first. Yet in reality, women are 'created' first. And, sorry to tell you this, guys, you're nothing more (or less) than modified women. Women gone wrong, some might say. However, here's a fascinating little piece of information to bolster the male ego. Every egg and every sperm contains a unique assortment of chromosomes, but whereas women only ever produce perhaps 500 unique eggs, men produce 425 billion unique sperm cells in a lifetime. Now that really takes some doing!

Men are just women gone wrong

Men and women think of themselves as very different, and in the matter of sex they see themselves as opposites. In fact, male and female embryos are anatomically identical during the first weeks of development. At six to seven weeks, the foetus looks essentially female with no external genitals other than a tiny protuberance called the 'genital tubercle'. Inside will be two primitive gonads. If the egg was fertilized by a sperm carrying an X chromosome, the foetus will continue to develop as a female, the gonads will become ovaries and the genital tubercle will become the clitoris. But if the egg was fertilized by a sperm carrying a Y chromosome, the foetus will be flooded with male hormones, the gonads will become testes, and the genital tubercle will become the head, or glans, of the penis.

Four weeks after that first flooding, a second flooding will alter the development of the brain. Very occasionally, a foetus is somehow resistant to one of the floodings – a condition known as Androgen Insensitivity Syndrome (AIS) – leading to the phenomenon of a male brain trapped in a woman's body or of a female brain trapped in a man's body.

In other words, a man's sex organs are derived from the same tissues as a woman's, as Table 1 below shows.

Table 1 Sex organs from the same embryonic tissue.

Men	Women
Testes	Ovaries
Penis	Clitoral system
Penile glans	Clitoral glans
Foreskin	Clitoral hood
Scrotum	Labia majora
Cowper's glands	Bartholin's glands

Apart from being a rather entertaining thought, this means that men and women are not really so very different after all. The things you discover about your own body can, to a degree, also be applied to your partner's body. At one time it was thought that women couldn't have orgasms in the way that men could. Now we know differently. And at one time it was thought men couldn't have multiple orgasms as women could. Now we know differently.

Great masturbation

Men need very little encouragement to masturbate. Even in Alfred Kinsey's day, over 90 per cent of men sometimes masturbated. A later *Playboy* survey found that almost three-quarters of men were still masturbating after marriage. My guess is that just about all men masturbate, irrespective of age and whether or not they're in a relationship. Men should masturbate for the same reasons that women should masturbate, but with two differences. Few men have any problem reaching orgasm, but they do have to learn how to control orgasm and ejaculation. This is vital to great sex and essential for multiple orgasms (see Chapter 8). Moreover, when a man doesn't have regular sex with a partner, masturbation is beneficial to the prostate and may help prevent prostate cancer.

12 GREAT REASONS WHY MEN SHOULD MASTURBATE

1 *Masturbation teaches you how to control orgasm.*
2 *Masturbation relieves tension.*
3 *Masturbation helps to develop your sexual responsiveness.*
4 *Masturbation teaches you about your own body.*
5 *Masturbation helps you to learn techniques in private before trying with a partner.*
6 *Masturbation helps you to understand your partner's body.*
7 *Masturbation provides the sexual activity vital to mental and physical health when no partner is available.*
8 *Masturbation makes you happy.*
9 *Masturbation is readily available.*
10 *Masturbation is free.*
11 *Masturbation is safe.*
12 *Masturbation is good for the prostate when no partner is available.*

Insight

There are going to be times when you'd really like to be able to masturbate while you're making love to your partner. When you don't immediately get a strong erection, for example, or when your erection goes down, or when you'd like to continue intercourse after ejaculating and you need some really strong stimulation to get going again. So try to get comfortable with the idea of masturbating when you're with your partner. Your partner also needs to be comfortable with the idea of you stimulating yourself during lovemaking. She can masturbate, too, of course.

I hope I've demonstrated that there's no need to feel guilty about masturbation. Use it for pleasure but also use it for practice. Before you can really enjoy great sex with a partner, you need to explore great sex on your own. Only when you know your own body can you guide your partner in the things that please you. And, amazing as it may seem, your body is far more like your partner's than you ever imagined. The touches that excite you are often just the same as those that will excite her.

Some men just use their fingers and hands to masturbate. Others use a vibrator or artificial vagina (see Chapter 9). Some like a vibrator in the anus as well. Still others make a vagina by, for example, cutting a hole in a melon. Fantasies, pictures and films can all be used to increase excitement. Be inventive. That's one of the things that makes for great sex. Don't always go for quick relief. Take the time to explore your whole body. Try stimulating different places as detailed below. If a place which you know is erogenous in others isn't erogenous in you, spend some time on it regularly. The aim is to awaken the sensuality of as many parts of your body as possible.

Men's 'bits'

This section details all of a man's important 'bits', but excluding the mind, which is dealt with in Chapter 7.

THE PENIS

The penis is essentially three parallel tubes of spongy tissue. The tube on the underside (the side that in the flaccid state, hangs against the testicles) is known as the 'corpus spongiosum'. It is the smallest of the three and surrounds the urethra, the tube that carries semen and urine. The other two, the 'corpora cavernosa', are located above the corpus spongiosum, and side by side. The tissues of all three tubes are a mass of tiny compartments. Sexual excitement causes a widening of these compartments as well as a widening of the arteries supplying blood to the penis. At the same time, valves limit the return of blood out of the penis. The result is an erection.

The tip of the penis is known as the 'glans', the underside of which creates particularly pleasurable sensations. To protect this delicate area, men have a foreskin, unless they've been circumcised. The widest part of the glans is known as the 'coronal ridge'. Even when the penis is apparently fully erect there's still a little extra enlargement in the coronal ridge area just prior to ejaculation. The little strip of skin attached to the glans on the underside is known as the 'frenulum' and may also create extreme pleasure. The rest of the penis is known as the 'shaft', of which the dark line underneath is the best bit. The amount of pleasure the penis creates for its owner is generally proportionate to the degree of erection.

A lot of men are concerned about the size of their penises. Nobody really knows what the average length is in erection but the widely accepted figure is around 14 cm (5.5 inches). As we saw in the previous chapter, even an excited vagina only measures 10 cm – 4 inches – (and has to stretch to accommodate anything longer), of which only the first 2.5 cm (1 inch) is very sensitive. Therefore, length doesn't matter physically. If you have a short penis, there are techniques and positions that can still give both you and your partner incredible pleasure (see Chapters 5 and 6). Penises that are small in repose have a proportionately greater increase in size than larger penises. Some women might be excited by the idea of a large penis, but many others actually prefer a shorter one. If you're dissatisfied with the length of your penis in erection, then you might like to try the exercises in Chapter 14.

Hygiene and the penis

A substance called 'smegma', composed of oily secretions, sweat, dead skin, dirt and bacteria, can collect between the foreskin and the glans. To prevent it, wash daily as well as before sex.

Facts about the penis

▶ *The interval between contractions is 0.8 seconds during orgasm.*
▶ *The penis has three to ten penile contractions during orgasm.*
▶ *The average duration of orgasm is four seconds.*
▶ *Six is the typical number of erections during sleep.*
▶ *Although there are internet accounts of men ejaculating huge distances, the pioneering sex researcher Alfred Kinsey proved that in the majority of men semen only seeps out.*
▶ *40.2 km (25 mph) is the maximum speed of ejaculation.*

Have a go

See how long you can stimulate yourself – enough to maintain an erection but without ejaculating. Next time try to double it. And then double it again. Good control is essential if you want to explore multiple orgasms (see Chapter 8).

Tips for women

A penis needs lubrication just as much as a vagina. While the penis is flaccid it isn't very sensitive to sexual pleasure but it can still hurt and needs to be treated gently. Once erect, the penis can be treated with more pressure. Find out where your partner's penis is most sensitive. Usually it's the frenulum side of the glans and the frenulum itself. Don't have sex with a man who has smegma – make sure he washes his penis first.

THE TESTICLES

The testicles, or testes, have two functions, to produce hormones and to produce sperm, and they continue doing both until a man dies. The hormones, notably testosterone, are made in the 'Leydig cells', while sperm are produced in tightly coiled microscopic tubes called 'seminiferous tubules'.

The scrotum, which contains the testicles, is more than a sack of loose skin. It has muscle fibres that contract to draw the testicles closer to the body during sexual excitement (and in cold weather). The muscle fibres relax in warm weather to keep the testicles cool.

Facts about the testicles
▶ *If the seminiferous tubules were stretched out to their fullest extent they would measure 500 m (1,640.5 ft).*
▶ *The entire process of sperm production takes 70 days.*
▶ *The average amount of semen ejaculated by a man in a lifetime is 45 litres (10 gallons).*
▶ *The average number of sperm ejaculated by a man in a lifetime is 425 billion.*

Have a go
See what happens when you tickle your testicles, stroke them and squeeze them. If anything nice happens, tell your partner.

Tips for women
Once aroused, most men enjoy having their scrotums caressed during sex.

THE PERINEUM

The area between the anus and the testicles is known as the 'perineum' and once you're aroused it will probably feel very nice to stroke it. About half way along there's a small area where a finger can sink in. In acupressure it's known as 'Inner Meeting' and in sex as the 'Million dollar point'. Some sexologists recommend pressing it hard to indirectly stimulate the prostate gland and to interrupt ejaculation. My own opinion is that it's ineffective at stimulating the prostate and potentially harmful when used for controlling ejaculation. I'll be showing you better ways of doing both.

Have a go
When excited, see what kinds of caress are enjoyable on the perineum.

Tips for women

When you're next having sex with your partner, try caressing the perineum and see what happens. Using lubricant will almost certainly enhance the effect.

THE ANUS

During ejaculation the anus contracts two to four times (except after the age of 50 or so when it stops reacting). And just like a woman's, a man's anus is absolutely packed with nerve endings. In fact, when a man is already highly excited a little stimulation here can easily tip him over into orgasm. The anus also provides a pathway to the prostate gland, which in women, as we've seen, is accessed via the G-spot. So, guys, learn to love your anus and, if you don't already, include it in masturbation and love play.

Insight

Some men fear that if they get to like anal stimulation it must mean that they're homosexual or are encouraging homosexual tendencies in themselves. There's absolutely no truth in that at all.

The anatomy of a man's anal canal and rectum is exactly the same as that for a woman, as already described. The key point to understand is that there's never any waste matter in the anal canal, nor will there be any in the rectum for some time after it's been emptied. It goes without saying that any activity involving the anus and rectum calls for scrupulous hygiene and an absolute certainty that there's no risk of spreading disease. Anything that's been inserted into the anus must be thoroughly washed before anything else is done with it.

Have a go

Once you're already excited, explore your anus. Lubricate a forefinger and run it along the 'gully' between your buttocks. Try circling movements on the anus itself. If it feels nice, insert your lubricated finger until the first joint. Experiment

(Contd)

with different effects, such as twisting the finger to stroke the highly sensitive wall of the anal canal, moving it in and out, and increasing the feeling of openness by adding a second finger. While masturbating your penis you should notice that anal penetration increases the excitement. Deeper penetration is dealt with below, under 'The prostate'. You can also experiment with anal vibrators.

Tips for women

Like your own anus (with which you're hopefully now familiar), your partner's anus needs plenty of lubrication, otherwise anything you do won't be pleasurable and might even be painful. During sex, try reaching around and slipping a lubricated fingertip into his anus. You should immediately notice an increase in his excitement. Don't worry about anal penetration being messy. There's never any waste matter in the anal canal, which is longer than your fingertip can reach.

THE PROSTATE

The prostate gland is a vital part of the male sexual apparatus. One of its roles is to contribute prostatic fluid to the semen, and the more it can be encouraged to produce, the longer ejaculation can continue. What's more, its contractions contribute to the pleasurable feelings of orgasm. Consequently, the prostate is one of the keys to great sex.

The prostate encircles the urethra, like a tiny doughnut, well inside the body just below the bladder. At first sight, then, it isn't easy to stimulate. But, in fact, there is a way. Some sexologists say it can be excited via the Million dollar point on the perineum, described above, but in my opinion that's pretty ineffective and even potentially harmful. It's also possible to exert some pressure by contracting the PC muscle, once it's been trained (see page 56). But the finest way is to insert a finger through the anus and well into the rectum as described below in 'Have a go'. Stimulation of the prostate should feel very nice and will, if continued, cause some liquid to be expelled from the penis. Men over 50, however, might not feel very much from direct prostate stimulation, although the anal penetration should continue to be exciting.

Have a go

The first step is to locate the prostate. As it lies about 5.5 cm (2.25 inches) from the anus, you'll have to insert your finger up to the second joint, with the pad facing towards your navel. Now press on the wall of the rectum. Don't curl your finger. You'll know if you're on the prostate because it feels quite distinct and is about the size of a grape (although it could be much larger if you're past 50). If you can't identify it as something quite separate from the surrounding tissue, then you're not on it. The final test is to keep your finger there while you masturbate to ejaculation. You'll feel the prostate contract several times. Don't confuse the contractions with the pulsation of the blood vessel there. You'll know the difference by the fact that the blood keeps on pumping once the ejaculation is over, although less forcefully, whereas the prostate doesn't.

Tips for women

It's probably a good idea to become familiar with your own anus and rectum before exploring your partner's. The best time to stimulate his prostate is while masturbating him or during intercourse, especially with him squatting between your legs in the improved missionary position, thus providing easy access (see Chapter 6). If you have small fingers, you may have to insert your forefinger all the way to locate his prostate, rather than just to the second joint. Once you go beyond the anal canal you might encounter waste matter. He should know what the chance of that is and, if necessary, suggest you defer direct prostate stimulation to another session. If you don't want to go in as far as the rectum, stimulating the anal canal as described above is a pretty good substitute. Don't forget the lubrication.

THE PC MUSCLE

We've already learned about a woman's PC muscle in Chapter 2. A man has one too, and it's just as important because, among other things, the stronger it is, the stronger a man's orgasms will be.

The PC muscle runs from the pubic bone to the spine, passing immediately under the prostate gland and, by flexing it, a man can give himself a prostate massage, as mentioned above. If you're not really aware of your PC muscle, try stopping the flow of urine next time you urinate. *That's* the muscle. If you can't do it even once, then your PC muscle is weak.

Exercising and strengthening the PC muscle is one of the keys to great sex. Insert a lubricated finger into your rectum as far as it will go and try contracting your PC. You should notice that the pressure on your finger begins at the base and continues up to your fingertip the harder you squeeze. At the level of your fingertip, the PC will be working on your prostate gland.

Have a go
Exercise your PC muscle every day. You can contract it quite invisibly whenever you want – while you're watching television, for example. A full exercise programme for the PC is given in Chapter 11.

Tips for women
Remind your partner to do his PC exercises – perhaps while you're doing yours.

THE HEAD

Eyes

Most books on sex neglect to mention a man's eyes as important sexual organs. In fact, they're probably *the* most important organs for arousal.

Women don't tend to get as excited by visual sensation as men (although there's a cultural element to this that seems to be changing) so a woman can be quite mystified by her partner's behaviour. Try to remember that for men to use porn films or pictures of naked women as props for masturbation is entirely normal. It's also quite normal for men to have particular visual triggers such as, say, black underwear or a suspender belt. This isn't fetishism unless he can't get excited without them.

Nose

Men tend to find the perfume of women's vulvas rather exciting. So much so that some men prefer their partners not to wash too much. What's more, when they masturbate, men quite like that vulval perfume to help them get aroused. Which brings us to the laundry basket. Girls, if you've ever opened yours and thought the contents were arranged differently to the way you left them, it's probably because your man has been rummaging around in there looking for your underwear.

And yet exactly what it is about a woman's natural scent is somewhat controversial. One body of opinion holds that we all produce chemical signals known as pheromones, just as so many other creatures do, and that those pheromones can be detected by a tiny area well inside the nose, known as the 'vomeronasal organ' or VNO. Other scientists say the VNO no longer functions in modern humans and that men can't detect women's pheromones, if they exist. The problem isn't easily resolved because pheromones don't necessarily have any 'smell' as such and experiments with pheromone-enhanced perfumes have given patchy results.

My own opinion, for what it's worth, is that women *do* produce pheromones and that men *can* detect them. But even if that isn't the case, the fact remains that men find the scent of a vulva exciting.

Ears
Biting, sucking and blowing in a man's ears can be effective. 'Talking dirty' in them even more so.

Neck
Most men aren't as interested in kissing as women are but his neck is certainly worth trying.

Tongue
For extra stimulation suck and bite his tongue.

Have a go
Try to find out how susceptible you are to pheromones. If you've ever found yourself becoming excited for no apparent reason, pheromones could be the explanation. If your partner is willing to co-operate, see how you react to her just before and just after a bath.

Tips for women
Try to get used to the idea that your partner could become aroused by the pheromones you produce. If you're squeamish about it, then try not to be. Millions of years of evolution have gone into this and it's no different, in principle, to his being attracted by the way you look or the things you say.

ALL THE OTHER BITS

In general, men's breasts and nipples aren't as sensitive as women's. Some men become sexually aroused when their nipples are stroked, and others feel very little. In about half of men the nipples become erect during sex.

Men are not generally as responsive on their skin as women either so it may take a little slapping and biting to get a reaction. If he's been naughty, take a slipper to his buttocks.

Have a go
While masturbating, explore the less erogenous areas of your body. If anything nice happens, tell your partner. Try caressing your breasts and nipples. In my focus groups, some men have said that they've 'taught' their nipples to be responsive in this way.

Tips for women
Very light touches can be interesting, but your man will probably need stronger stimulation than you would.

TEN THINGS EVERY WOMAN SHOULD KNOW ABOUT A MAN

1 *The most sensitive part of the penis is the glans (the bit at the top), especially the frenulum side (the side with the little cleft in it); the rest varies in sensitivity from man to man and also depends on the degree of erection.*
2 *Men need lubrication on the penis just as much as women do in the vagina, otherwise stimulation just hurts.*
3 *After ejaculation men experience a 'refractory' period during which they cannot have any more sex; the period lasts from a few minutes in some young men up to hours in the case of older men.*
4 *Some men are capable of ejaculating several times a day; other men only one or two times a week.*
5 *You need to have your orgasms before and at the same time as your partner ejaculates because, unless he's unusual, he won't be giving you any more orgasms afterwards.*
6 *Men can enjoy non-penetrative sex just as much as women.*
7 *Almost all men masturbate.*
8 *Almost all men enjoy pornography.*

9   It's normal for men to be excited by the perfume of a woman's vulva.
10 Men sometimes do have headaches – stress and overwork can lead to loss of interest in sex.

What happens during orgasm and ejaculation?

If, like most men, you use the words orgasm and ejaculation interchangeably then you're making a very common mistake:

▶ It's possible to ejaculate without having an orgasm.
▶ It's possible to orgasm without ejaculating.

Up until only a few years ago, Western scientists considered the two words to mean precisely the same thing, but Oriental thought has always separated them. Orgasm is the muscular contraction, and ejaculation is the passage of semen, and the two *can* take place separately.

I'm not going to say any more about this particular point now because it's the key to multiple orgasms for men, which is the subject of Chapter 8. What I want to examine here is exactly what happens during the whole process of orgasm and ejaculation, which is the usual climax to sex.

As with women, the whole sexual experience can be divided into four phases:

1   Excitement phase (when sexual tension builds rapidly).
2   Plateau phase (in which the tension is maintained or continues to grow slowly).
3   Orgasm (which releases the tension).
4   Resolution phase (in which things gradually return to normal).

However, unlike women, most men can experience the plateau and orgasm phases only once during a single lovemaking session.

During sexual excitement, two particular things happen:

▶ *vasocongestion*
▶ *myotonia.*

These are the technical words used by sexologists to describe changes in the body with which we're all familiar. 'Vasocongestion' is simply the build-up of blood in the pelvic area, especially in the penis (about a quarter of men also develop a sex flush of the skin). Here again there is a difference with women. Erection of the penis takes a mere three to eight seconds (longer in older men), and although vasocongestion goes on building for a time, it doesn't increase over hours as it can in women. In other words, men are quicker to become fully aroused.

A few drops of fluid from the Cowper's glands may appear at the tip of the penis almost straight away. These drops contain sperm, and although some scientists say the sperm are not viable, women have become pregnant through overenthusiastic foreplay; if a condom is being used for contraception, it must be put on before there's any contact at all between the penis and the vulva.

'Myotonia' simply means increased muscular tension. This can happen all over the body and is why we all pull faces when excitement rises. It's partly involuntary and partly voluntary.

These reactions and lots of others (including breathing rate, heart rate, blood pressure, elevation of the testicles and, in about half of all men, nipple erection) are controlled more or less by the same chemicals as for women. Prolactin particularly should be mentioned because it's the chemical that stops you having one ejaculation straight after another.

Climax is the release of the muscular tension, and in men this occurs in broadly three stages:

▶ **Stage one.** *The various fluids that compose the semen build up; at this point ejaculation isn't inevitable.*

▸ **Stage two.** *The fluids mix in a wide part of the urethra known as the bulb, which is located at the base of the penis. This is the point of no return (PNR); in other words, ejaculation is inevitable.*

▸ **Stage three.** *Ejaculation.*

If you want to experience multiple orgasms, it's important that you learn to recognize the approach of stage two. This is separated from ejaculation by a short interval. In young men this interval may be as long as three seconds, which can be enough to allow a highly aroused woman to respond by commencing an orgasm of her own. In older men, however, there may be almost no separation between stage two and ejaculation; as a result the man is taken by surprise and the woman has no time to respond. Young or old, once the PNR has passed, the semen is fired out of the penis by the combined contractions of the prostate, urethra, penis and PC muscle. In men under the age of 50 or so, the anus also contracts.

Yet why does orgasm feel so nice? Because there's also a sort of 'orgasm' in the brain. Not a physical spasm in this case, but a release of 'happy' chemicals, which I've already detailed in Chapter 2 on women's bodies. These chemicals make simultaneous orgasm so special. If you don't orgasm together, one of you will be wanting to go to sleep while the other is still in a state of tension. If you do orgasm together, you'll both experience bliss. How this is achieved is explained in Chapter 6.

....

Insight

Many men find the pleasure of ejaculation is related to frequency. When they haven't been having much sex of any kind, they become excited too quickly and ejaculate too easily, with little sense of tension or release. On the other hand, when they've been ejaculating too often, the next ejaculation can become a desperate struggle. The perfect frequency is when there's that sense of the ejaculate being drawn up from the back of the knees. Try to discover your own optimum frequency of ejaculation and stick to it.

But didn't I say you should have sex as frequently as possible? Yes, I did, but as you'll see in Chapter 8, you don't have to ejaculate to have sex!

TECHNIQUES FOR DEFERRING ORGASM AND EJACULATION

When masturbating, women are on average capable of reaching orgasm almost as quickly as men (in some cases faster). But that's not the same thing as reaching maximum arousal. When you're making love with your partner, you don't want to orgasm too quickly because she'll be wanting to get as close as possible to that maximum state. Apart from which, it makes sense to prolong your own pleasure as much as possible, a subject I'll be covering in detail in Chapter 8. In the meantime, here are some basic techniques to practise. Don't expect to perfect them in one session. Keep trying and see which one works best for you

Stop/go
You probably already use stop/go. It simply means that instead of rushing to orgasm/ejaculation as quickly as possible, you cease stimulation once you begin to get too excited. After things have calmed down a bit you resume. Try varying the length of the 'rest period' from a few seconds up to a minute or more. See how many times you can do it before you 'have' to orgasm.

Imsak
An extreme form of stop/go, *imsak* involves withdrawing completely from the vagina and cooling off for a bit before resuming. It's a traditional Arab technique from a word meaning 'retention' and those who are expert at it re-enter up to ten times before ejaculating (see Chapter 5).

Mind control
This again uses the physical technique of stop/go, but adds in the mental resolve not to ejaculate for a predetermined length of time. (It helps to have a clock somewhere you can easily see it.)

The locking method
First described by the physicians of the Chinese Taoist religion thousands of years ago, it consists quite simply of contracting the PC and abdominal muscles at the same time, so that the stomach is pulled as tightly back towards the spine as possible. Do it each time you start to get excited. Also try holding the muscles contracted while continuing stimulation. During intercourse this is particularly easy to do when the woman is in a rear-entry position and the man is on his knees.

The panting method
When you get close to the PNR stop what you're doing, let your tongue hang out and pant.

The squeeze method
The squeeze method was developed by the sex scientists William Masters and Virginia Johnson to help men who ejaculate prematurely. Personally, I don't consider it of much value but I'm including it because it might work for you. The idea is to use the squeeze intermittently as often as necessary well before the PNR. There are two versions. For the first, squeeze the base of the shaft of the penis, from front to back, using the thumb and two fingers, for around four seconds. For the second, the man's partner puts her thumb on the frenulum with her first and second fingers on the opposite side of the penis, one just above and one just below the coronal ridge. She then squeezes firmly, also for about four seconds. My own opinion is that going without stimulation for a few seconds will decrease excitement anyway, while pressure on the glans might even increase the likelihood of ejaculating.

The testicle pull
Because the testicles move up closer to the body just before ejaculation some sexologists advise that the reverse – pulling the testicles down – must prevent ejaculation. This is another method I don't personally think much of but you might find it works in your case. Be gentle, otherwise the pain will certainly call at least a temporary halt to things.

Remember none of these are techniques for stopping the semen once ejaculation has commenced. Exponents of the Million dollar point, previously mentioned, claim they can do this but I consider the technique potentially harmful and would not recommend it.

Tips for women
If your partner is practising the various techniques for retarding ejaculation while making love to you, it may make for a rather disrupted session. Try to go along with it – it's all in a good cause.

THE KEYS TO GREAT EJACULATIONS

To recap, then, the keys to great ejaculations are:

▶ *a healthy body and a healthy diet (because those chemicals don't come out of nowhere)*
▶ *time to build up vasocongestion and myotonia*
▶ *stimulation of the prostate gland, directly or indirectly*
▶ *a strong PC muscle.*

THE MALE CYCLE

Women have a monthly cycle and men have a rather different one, driven by the frequency of sex. As we've seen, sex causes changes in the levels of certain hormones including dopamine, PEA, oxytocin, serotonin and prolactin. Another hormone is testosterone, the 'male sex hormone'.

Between 6 and 8 mg of testosterone are produced per day, mostly in the testes but with a tiny additional amount from the adrenal glands. (What most men probably don't know is that they also produce oestrogen, the 'female sex hormone'.) In the right quantity, testosterone is a hugely beneficial hormone, but too much or too little can lead to all kinds of problems, including personality disorders.

Some men have higher base levels of testosterone than others, but every man's level is constantly changing. It's actually the part of the brain called the 'hypothalamus' that measures the level of testosterone in the blood. If it's too high or too low, the hypothalamus sends a message to the pituitary gland, which in turn sends a message to the testes. However, it seems that in each individual the hypothalamus accepts a wide ranging testosterone level, which fluctuates according to various factors including temperature, health, stress, alcohol use … and sexual activity.

Quite simply, changes in the level of testosterone and other hormones mean that men quite genuinely feel more appreciative when they want sex but some time after sex feel less appreciative and can even become irritable and aggressive. How long after sex depends on age and various other factors. This is known as the 'sexual hangover' and in Chapter 10 you will see how you can stop it spoiling your great sex.

10 THINGS TO REMEMBER

1 *Men and women aren't really so very different because men effectively begin their lives in the womb as females.*

2 *Masturbation is essential to the development of sexual skills.*

3 *Pleasure isn't related to penis size but to technique.*

4 *The testicles produce sperm and the male sex hormone testosterone.*

5 *The anus is so packed with nerve endings that stimulating it can make a man ejaculate.*

6 *Stimulating the prostate gland can increase the volume of ejaculate.*

7 *The strength of the PC muscle, which is involved in orgasm and ejaculation, can be increased with exercise.*

8 *Orgasm and ejaculation are not the same thing.*

9 *Techniques for delaying ejaculation include stop/go, the squeeze method, the Million dollar point and the locking method, but none of these prevents ejaculation once the point of no return (PNR) has been passed.*

10 *Like women, men have a hormonal cycle, but theirs is based on the pattern of sexual activity.*

HOW GREAT IS SEX NOW?

▶ *Have you been masturbating more frequently and more happily?*   Yes/No

▶ *Have you extended the time you can masturbate without ejaculating?*   Yes/No

▶ *Have you masturbated together with your partner?*   Yes/No

▶ *Have you tried stimulating your anus during masturbation?*   Yes/No

▶ *Have you located your prostate gland?*   Yes/No

▶ *Have you identified your PC muscle and begun exercising it?*   Yes/No

▶ *Have you learned to recognize your point of no return (PNR)?*   Yes/No

▶ *Have you experimented with the techniques for delaying ejaculation? (Which one worked best?)*   Yes/No

▶ *Have you discovered your optimum frequency of ejaculation?*   Yes/No

If you answered 'no' to more than three questions, re-read the relevant parts of the chapter and make an effort to put the suggestions into effect. Think of masturbation not only as pleasure but also as training. Understanding and controlling your own body is an essential prelude to great sex with a partner.

4

Great opening moves

In this chapter you will learn:
- *how to initiate sex*
- *how to arouse your partner even without touching*
- *how to create the perfect atmosphere for sex.*

Great sex doesn't start when you get into bed. It doesn't even start 30 minutes before you get into bed. In fact, it never really stops. Great sex should be all the time. In other words, let's suppose the sexual buzz between you and your partner could be measured on a scale from zero up to 100, which would be orgasm. Never let things drop to zero. That's far too much of a climb back up. When you're not actually in bed together, keep things oscillating between, say, 30 and 50. Or, to put it another way, don't just be nice to your partner when you want sex.

Keeping the sexual temperature up

Remember how it was when you first fell in love? You had that walking on air feeling because your body was powered by phenylethylamine (PEA). Nothing else mattered but the two of you. However, over time, it's true, things can change. The PEA level goes down. You have a job, a career plan, shelves to put up, a lawn to mow, maybe children, maybe grandchildren. You still love your partner, but other things matter too. And, then, there are all those little resentments that have developed. The wounds that are still tender and can't take any more hurt.

Once it was so easy. You just began kissing. Or putting your hands somewhere. There was never any question of *not* having sex. Now, perhaps, there is. It's 'Yes, but I'm busy right now.' 'I'm exhausted.' 'I've got to be at such and such by seven o'clock.' And that can hurt. Rejection is very hard to take. Many people respond by simply giving up trying. That way, they don't have to face rejection any more. With less sex comes more resentment. You're on a downwards spiral.

If this sounds a little like you, what can you do about it? The first step is to return your relationship to the way it was when nothing was more important. Because nothing *is* more important. Your love affair has to be 24 hours a day, 7 days a week, 365 days a year, *not* 30 minutes twice a week.

Some experts say that the PEA effect only lasts for a few months. Others say the maximum is two years. Almost everyone agrees that no relationship can remain exciting for long. Well, it can. This book explains how.

If you actually have to seduce your partner every time, that is, overcome resistance, then something's wrong. You *have* to find out what it is. You *have* to communicate. You *have* to put it right.

Here are some of the reasons that people give for no longer behaving as they did when they first fell in love:

- ▶ *It's ridiculous to behave like a couple of silly teenagers. Why is it?*
- ▶ *She or he doesn't deserve it. You need to do some work on your relationship.*
- ▶ *I'd rather watch television/do the gardening/go shopping. You need to re-examine your priorities.*
- ▶ *Other people don't behave like that. Maybe not, but then again other people separate or get divorced.*

Here are some ideas for getting back to being 'silly teenagers':

- *Swap items of clothing and go to work in them. The more intimate the better.*
- *Send naughty text messages.*
- *Send flowers.*
- *When you shower, shower together; when you bath, bath together.*
- *When you read, sit back to back like bookends.*
- *Hold hands.*
- *Get T-shirts printed with personal messages.*
- *Talk dirty.*
- *If you have to be apart, have phone sex.*

Insight

If you really can't make time for one another, then you need to take a long, hard look at your lives to see how you can change them. Try making a list of the things in your life and put them in order of priority. Where does your relationship come? Where does sex come? Think about moving closer to work so that you commute less and have more time at home. If necessary, think about changing your job.

Make sex routine

I hesitate to use the word 'routine' when talking about great sex. Surely great sex should be something spontaneous and imaginative? The very opposite of routine? Yes, but what I'm getting at is that there should be a sort of presumption between you and your partner that you will have sex with a certain regularity. I suggest it should be *every day*.

Too much for you? Well, in reality, you probably won't achieve it anyway. In modern life there are so many things that intrude, without even mentioning heavy periods, illness, children, emergencies and so on. Let's say that by aiming to have sex every day you actually manage it every other day. Whereas if you aimed to have sex once a week you'd probably end up never doing it at all.

In my focus groups, some people said that daily sex would be 'boring'. Yet, curiously, nobody ever said daily eating would be 'boring'. And, in fact, after they'd tried daily sex for a while, they changed their minds. Their bodies got used to it. Some older men may think they just physically aren't capable, but they probably are (see Chapters 8 and 13).

When are you going to find the time? Well, on work days why not set the alarm a little earlier? Okay, most people don't feel very good on waking up. But have a cup of tea, freshen up and you're ready. Once you've had sex, the day ahead looks different. You're already off to a great start.

Then, in the evenings and at the weekends, *make* time. Many couples say they don't have time but they do, really. If lack of time is your excuse, do a little 'time and motion' study on your life. Maybe you could watch less television?

Wining and dining

Wining and dining is the traditional preliminary to a night of love. In fact, the whole idea probably goes back hundreds of thousands of years to when a man would have to prove he could be a good provider by dropping a mammoth's thigh by the fire. In the early days of a relationship, most women expect to be wined and dined. However, this is actually a very bad idea where sex is concerned. A full stomach is hardly conducive to anything even vaguely athletic and it can be quite uncomfortable. Furthermore, alcohol reduces sensation, which is the opposite of what you want. What's more, by the time you get back from the restaurant, you'll probably be exhausted anyway. Go for a meal afterwards, if you wish, but not before. Alternatively, use wining and dining as a way of making time to communicate with one another, not as an aphrodisiac. It just doesn't work.

> **Insight**
>
> Guys, don't get the idea that buying a meal entitles you to sex. It doesn't.

Pheromones

Everybody smells slightly different, which is why dogs are able to track people. As I already mentioned in Chapter 2, a surprising number of women in my focus groups said they found the smell of their partners arousing. I'm going to stick my neck out and join the group of scientists who say it's at least partly due to pheromones. It seems to me that men are easily excited by pheromones and that women are very good at producing them. And it seems to work the other way around just as well.

Pheromones, of course, are chemical messengers. Take the butterfly, for example. The male butterfly can detect the pheromones of an available female at a distance of as much as 1.6 km (1 mile). Human beings are nowhere near as sensitive, of course, and ever since the invention of language, pheromones have probably been diminishing in importance. But I'm sure they're still there. In fact, you wouldn't be consciously aware of pheromones because they have no identifiable smell, yet work they almost certainly do. When a woman is already sexually aroused she releases pheromones that can't fail to turn a man on, even if he himself doesn't realize what it is that's exciting him.

Therefore, if you want to invite your man into bed without saying a word, the best advice is not to wash *too much*. Otherwise you wash all the pheromones away. And if you think sexy thoughts the output of pheromones will undoubtedly increase. If you're a man and want to invite your woman into bed, see if you can find out exactly what it is about your smell that she likes.

Body language

Body language is another way of inviting your partner into bed
without actually saying anything. You can begin with subtle hints.
A look into the eyes. A raised eyebrow. If your partner is a little
too preoccupied to notice then you may have to be more obvious.
Women can do this far more successfully than men simply because
men are far more easily aroused by physical signals. A tongue run
around the lips, tilting the head back to run hands through hair
while the breasts are thrust forward, a dress slipping off a shoulder...

Insight

You can learn a thing or two from the films. Remember Faye
Dunaway sucking a chess piece in the original of *The Thomas
Crown Affair*? Or Sharon Stone in *Basic Instinct*?

Letters, texts and emails

Erotic text and email messages may seem like a modern invention,
but only the technology is new. In fact, the first words ever written
down were probably: 'My cave or yours?'

Some 'dirty' messages are of the subtle kind. Two hundred years
ago, for example, Nelson, that great British hero, was writing to
his lover Emma Hamilton of how he longed to visit her 'thatched
cottage' – his code for the pubic mound.

Gertrude Stein, writer of unreadable prose, wrote poems for her
lover Alice Babette Toklas, about the 'cow' that would be made to
'come out'. Huh? Apparently a cow was a euphemism for an orgasm.

MISSION IMPOSSIBLE

If writing isn't your thing, why not take a tip from the film *Mission
Impossible*? Leave a sexy message on a pocket voice recorder and

then telephone your partner with instructions on where to find it. Via the machine you can say all those things you've wanted to say but never dared to. Don't just record 'I'll be in the bedroom waiting for you at six o'clock.' Make it a little more exciting and inventive: 'Your mission is to excite me beyond anything that has ever been achieved before...' I'll leave the rest to you.

The power of touch

Almost 2,500 years ago, Hippocrates recognized the power of touch. Today, we know 'scientifically' that skin-to-skin contact changes the structure of the brain, transforms the outlook for severely deprived infants, and can even help heal certain diseases. Touch whenever you can. If you have children and they're around, there are still ways of doing this unobtrusively. When you look at other animal species, they touch all the time. Think of kittens sleeping on top of one another in a basket.

Make plenty of eye contact, too. Smile. We smile when we're happy, but smiling can also *make* us happy.

Insight

Kissing and cuddling are generally considered to be things that only women like. However, in my focus groups many men tell me they don't have enough physical affection from their partners. How can this be? A lot of women believe that men only offer cuddles when they want sex, and women resent that. Behind every cuddle they think they see an ulterior motive. There are two parts to the solution: better communication and a lot more cuddling.

GREAT CUDDLES

Cuddling is such a natural thing that it may seem silly to have formal positions for doing it. Nevertheless, we have special positions for intercourse and, in fact, when you cuddle in a way that has symmetry and harmony it can feel quite magical. The more skin contact the better.

In the descriptions that follow I'm assuming that the man is the tallest and heaviest. But, of course, there's no reason why a strong woman can't take the 'man's' role.

Cuddle 1: The human armchair
The man sits down with legs apart on somewhere comfortable like a bed or thickly carpeted floor. His back needs to be supported by, for example, a pile of pillows. The woman sits between his legs, facing the same way, and leaning back against him as if he's a nice comfortable armchair. In this position you can both read the same book or watch television together.

Cuddle 2: Sharing chairs
The woman sits on a chair and the man sits behind her on the same chair, with his arms around her.

Cuddle 3: The sitting embrace
The man sits cross-legged or with legs out straight. The woman then sits on his lap, facing him, with her legs crossed behind his back. It's a comfortable position in which you can embrace, kiss, co-ordinate breathing, and chat.

Cuddle 4: The human bed
The man lies face down somewhere soft and comfortable, and the woman lies on top, facing the same way, with her groin on his buttocks.

Cuddle 5: Spooning
Lie on your sides, facing the same way, each with one or both legs bent, so the buttocks of the person in front nestle in the groin of the person behind.

Cuddle 6: Full body contact
The man lies on his back and the woman lies on top, facing him. If you haven't got time to get naked then, at the very least, your feet should be naked and touching. (Even people in my focus groups

who *don't* believe in 'energy' flowing through and between bodies, say they notice a significant difference between feet touching and not touching.)

While you're cuddling you'll also be kissing, of course. Most men aren't very interested in prolonged sessions, but women like it a lot. It's worth practising and spending time over. Suck and gently bite one another's lips. Suck and gently bite one another's tongues – that's a powerful turn-on. Kiss, suck and bite the sides of the neck, the indentation of the chin, and the forehead just between the eyes. And don't forget to breathe into the ears now and then.

Insight

There's nothing like the touch of the sun to increase the libido, especially if you can sunbathe somewhere you can both be naked. Let the sun play between your legs.

MASSAGE

Massage is a great way of getting to know your partner's body, actually helping your partner to fight stress and illness and, of course, arousing him or her.

The subject of massage needs a book on its own. Better still, I recommend you to take a short course, say a weekend, to properly understand what you need to do (see 'Taking it further'). Meanwhile, here are some ideas to get you started.

A bed is too soft for a good massage. A folded blanket on the floor is much better. You'll need some kind of massage oil. Warm the oil first: a light oil from the kitchen, such as soya, grapeseed or almond, will do perfectly well. However, it's best not to use oil-based lubricants on a woman's genital area because they may encourage vaginal infections. Oil-based lubricants can also damage latex condoms. For the genitals, male or female, use water-based lubricants only.

The general principle is to work inwards from the hands and feet and upwards from the base of the spine. Ask your partner to tell you what feels good and what doesn't.

Techniques

▶ *'Effleurage' is the first technique, a French word denoting a soothing, stroking action. Try it on the back to begin with. Your partner should be laying face down, head turned sideways and arms down by their sides. With your hands covered in warm massage oil, put one hand each side of your partner's spine and push steadily up to the neck, keeping the whole surface of your hands and fingers in contact. When you arrive at the neck, continue out along the shoulders and then, with very light pressure only, glide your hands back down along your partner's sides to the starting position. Repeat several times.*

▶ *Kneading is a technique to use on tense muscles. The shoulders are a great place to start. At the end of effleurage, move both hands to one shoulder, pick up the muscle in one hand, squeeze it gently, then push it towards the other hand. The new hand then also kneads the muscle before pushing it back. In this way, the muscle is worked rhythmically between the two hands. Once you've done one shoulder, turn your attention to the other.*

▶ *Two fingers (the pads of your index and middle fingers) can be used to make small circular movements. Work your way up from the base of the spine to the neck, doing both sides simultaneously. You can also work on the muscles.*

If the massage is a prelude to more sexual action, you'll probably want to work out a programme that occasionally tantalizes the genitals and finally ends there with stimulation of the penis or clitoris. You could work first of all on the back and shoulders using all three techniques, then move to *effleurage* on the backs of the legs followed by kneading of the thighs and buttocks, then have your partner turn over for *effleurage* on the front of the legs. If you've done a good job, she or he should now be highly aroused.

Insight

The sexiest way to give a massage is to strip naked, put the massage oil on *yourself*, then rub yourself all over your partner's body. This is how it's done in the more erotic versions of the Japanese *nuru* ('slippery') massage, which

uses a gel made from seaweed. But massage oil or cream will
do almost as well – have your partner lay on an old sheet so
your bedding doesn't get spoilt.

Insight

Have you ever noticed that sometimes after exercise you
feel you want to make love? What happens is that the
hypothalamus part of the brain produces chemicals that
act like morphine. And, in fact, they're some of the same
chemicals that are produced during sex. Scientists call
these chemicals 'endorphins' (from combining the words
'endogenous', meaning 'produced naturally by the body', and
'morphine'). Essentially, the exercise is like the early stages
of lovemaking and, naturally, you now want to carry on
to a climax.

How much exercise does it take? Well, not too little but, then
again, not so much that you're tired. Running briskly for
around 30 minutes should do it. This will more than double
the endorphins in your blood. Or what about swimming to a
deserted beach, kayaking to an uninhabited island or cycling
to a secluded picnic spot?

Atmosphere

The right kind of ambience is important for great sex. This seems
to matter more to most women than to most men but it matters to
both sexes all the same.

SHOWERS AND BATHS

Baths aren't very good places for having sex or as a prelude to sex.
The warm water tends to make you sleepy and if it's over hot it can
make you feel dizzy or sick. Prolonged immersion wrinkles the skin
and dries the vagina. Better to take a shower together. Showers are
invigorating and are good places for sex. If you have a removable

shower head, you can squirt one another in some interesting ways, soap one another in some interesting places, and enjoy penetration in some interesting positions. It helps to have a large shower and something to hold on to.

> ## Insight
> Some men swear by cold showers as a way of having a second orgasm/ejaculation; possibly by driving blood away from the skin more becomes available to the penis. Why not give it a try?

MUSIC

Choose music with care. The right music can put both of you in the mood and is worth half an hour of kissing and caressing. More than that, music also influences the *style* of sex. Once you become excited you may no longer even be consciously aware of the music but it will direct your movements nonetheless. The music could be fast and furious. It could be languid. It could be delicate and sensitive. It could be romantic. It could be raunchy. Discuss the music beforehand or take turns to choose it. Classical concertos and symphonies are excellent because they're long and they build to a climax. If classical music isn't your thing, try compiling your own album of singles. For example:

▶ *dreamy – 'Gymnopédies' by Erik Satie*
▶ *mystical – Violin concerto 'The Leeds' by Howard Blake*
▶ *spiritual – 'Symphony No. 2' by Gustav Mahler*
▶ *smoochie – Diana Krall*
▶ *vigorous – 'Romanza' by Andrea Bocelli*
▶ *wild – Russian Gypsy Soul*
▶ *manic – 'Ride Of The Valkyries' by Richard Wagner*
▶ *Kama Sutra – Raghunath Manet*
▶ *fun – your own compilation of pop classics such as 'How Deep Is Your Love?' (Bee Gees) and 'I'm Not In Love' (10 CC).*

SCENTS

We've already talked about pheromones and the fact that everybody has a unique smell. However, that only works close up and personal. If you want to create the right atmosphere in a whole room you need something a little stronger. Burning joss sticks/incense can be good. Try them out beforehand – some have a cheap smell that is actually a turn-off whereas others have a musky aroma that many find extremely arousing.

LIGHTING

Not many people look good naked in the glare of powerful lights and, apart from that, nobody wants a beam of light right in the eyes. So, use uplighters and soft mood lighting in preference to ceiling lights. Candles can be great, but make sure they're not in a place where they might get knocked over. Hanging candle lanterns are the best solution. They're safer than naked flames and they can cast beautiful shadows.

Some people don't like any lights at all. Occasionally, sex in the dark can be an interesting variation but it shouldn't be the way you habitually make love. You need to be able to look into one another's eyes, at least part of the time. Moreover, the sight of his partner's naked body is important for a man's arousal. Most women are less concerned by that but, nevertheless, love to see their partners' faces, smiles and twinkling eyes.

Contraception

Contraception is a big subject and couples should take expert advice and think carefully before deciding which of the many forms of contraception they want to use. Table 2 (see page 83) is only intended as a quick guide to contraception from the point of view of great sex. Don't forget that contraceptive methods can always be combined. Just because a woman is on the pill, for example, it doesn't mean she no longer has the right to insist that her partner wears a condom. A condom is highly effective against the transmission of HIV (human immunodeficiency virus) and some other venereal diseases (for more on this see Chapter 14). Even where there's no fear about illness, it can make sense to use a condom in combination with some other form of contraception for ultimate protection (for example, if the woman is using a diaphragm).

Some methods of contraception have a significant impact on enjoyment. The female condom undoubtedly reduces pleasure for both parties, but the male condom could actually enhance enjoyment for young couples. That's because condoms reduce sensitivity and help virile young men to continue longer without ejaculating. On balance, a couple may both experience greater satisfaction as a result. Many older men, by contrast, may have difficulty maintaining erection or ejaculating at all if they can't feel the vagina, skin to skin (but see Insight on 'gel charging', page 187, for a special technique).

Hormonal methods of contraception may, in some cases, affect libido – dramatically so if the side effects are severe. Methods with no negative impact on sexual enjoyment include vasectomy and female sterilization (provided there's no psychological problem afterwards).

I've talked about couples deciding on contraception but, of course, no one has the right to insist that a partner uses a form of contraception that could be harmful to health.

What do the reliability figures in Table 2 actually mean? Reliability of, say, 98 per cent sounds pretty impressive but, in fact, it isn't quite as good as it appears. It means that if 100 couples use that method of contraception for one year, two women will become pregnant. Over a 25-year period that's 50 women – half of all who are using it. So, if you really want to avoid worrying about pregnancy you need a method (or combination of methods) that is as close to 100 per cent as possible.

I've not included the rhythm method (only having sex at certain times of the month) nor *coitus interruptus* (withdrawal before ejaculation) in Table 2 because they don't work. Spermicides and spermicidal sponges should only be considered when fertility is known to be low because of age or a medical problem.

Table 2 Methods of contraception.

	For	Against	Great sex rating	Contraceptive reliability
Male condom	Although it reduces sensation, it can actually improve sex for young couples by extending the time the man can make love.	The lack of sensation may mean older men can't maintain an erection.	10/10 for pleasure for young couples, but this goes down sharply for older men; 9/10 for protection against disease.	98%
Female condom	Protects against disease as well as pregnancy.	Significant reduction in sensation for men and women; significant reduction in visual attraction for men.	0/10 for pleasure; 9/10 for protection against disease.	95%
The pill	Shorter, pain-free periods and no impairment to pleasure.	Health risks for certain women.	10/10 for pleasure; 0/10 for protection against disease.	Almost 100%
The mini-pill	Lower level of health risk than traditional pill.	Irregular periods.	10/10 for pleasure; 0/10 for protection against disease.	98%
Vasectomy	No health implications other than the minute risk of the surgery itself.	Nothing – as long as you're certain you don't want any more children.	10/10 for pleasure; 0/10 for protection against disease.	Almost 100% (failure rate is 1 in 2,000)

(Contd)

	For	Against	Great sex rating	Contraceptive reliability
Female sterilization	No health implications other than the small risk of the surgery itself.	Cost; you need to be certain you don't want any more children.	10/10 for pleasure; 0/10 for protection against disease.	99.5%
The contraceptive patch	You only have to apply one patch a week.	The patch might drop off without you noticing.	10/10 for pleasure; 0/10 for protection against disease.	99%
The contraceptive implant	Lasts about three years.	May cause depression and reduced libido.	10/10 for pleasure for some, but going down to 0/10 for those women who suffer from the side effects; 0/10 for protection against disease.	Almost 100%
The contraceptive injection	Lasts eight to 12 weeks.	May cause heavy, irregular periods and headaches (and the side effects could last until the injection has worn off).	10/10 for pleasure for some, but going down to 0/10 for those women who suffer from the side effects; 0/10 for protection against disease.	99%
The IUD – intrauterine device ('Coil')	No hormones involved.	Heavier, longer and more painful periods; some women suffer cramps on orgasm.	8/10 for pleasure; 0/10 for protection against disease.	98%

	For	Against	Great sex rating	Contraceptive reliability
The IUS – intrauterine system (Mirena)	Lasts five years and, after a few months, almost stops menstrual flow.	Nothing much.	10/10 for pleasure; 0/10 for protection against disease.	99%
The diaphragm and the cap	No hormones involved.	A bit tedious to insert (although this could be a sex game); may slip out of place.	9/10 for pleasure; 0/10 for protection against disease.	90–95%
Vaginal hormone ring (NuvaRing)	Only needs to be inserted once a month. Lower oestrogen exposure than some other hormonal methods.	14% of women in trials reported vaginal inflammation, 10% headaches, 6% discharge and 5% nausea. In susceptible women there might be an increased risk of blood clots and heart attacks.	9/10 for pleasure (the ring is flexible but might be felt during sex); 0/10 for protection against disease.	99%.

10 THINGS TO REMEMBER

1 *Keep the sexual temperature up all the time, not just ten minutes before you want sex.*

2 *Eliminate all reasons not to have sex.*

3 *Establish a presumption with your partner that you will have frequent sex.*

4 *Body language and pheromones can arouse your partner without any touching.*

5 *Write love letters and emails throughout your relationship.*

6 *Touch and cuddle whenever possible.*

7 *Exercise and sunshine are good ways of warming up to sex.*

8 *Learn how to give a good massage.*

9 *Establish the right atmosphere with lighting, music and scent.*

10 *Choose a contraceptive method that's effective and doesn't interfere with sexual enjoyment.*

HOW GREAT IS SEX NOW?

▶ *Have you been behaving like a silly teenager?*   Yes/No

▶ *Have you made sex a regular part of your routine?*   Yes/No

▶ *Have you increased your pheromone output?*   Yes/No

▶ *Have you been sending 'dirty' messages and making
  'dirty' phone calls?*   Yes/No

▶ *Have you increased the amount of cuddling?*   Yes/No

▶ *Have you given your partner a massage?*   Yes/No

▶ *Have you tried sex in the shower?*   Yes/No

▶ *Have you experimented with the effects of different
  kinds of music for making love?*   Yes/No

▶ *Have you got contraception expertly sorted out?*   Yes/No

If you answered 'no' to more than three questions, re-read the
relevant parts of the chapter and make an effort to put the
suggestions into effect. It's important to maintain a 'smoochy'
atmosphere all the time, not just when you want sex. Women,
understandably, tend to feel resentful if men only offer cuddles
when there's an ulterior motive, and the result is that they may
withdraw affection. Be romantic all the time – and, guys, that
especially applies to you.

5

Great sex techniques

In this chapter you will learn:
- *great warm-up techniques to use on yourself*
- *great techniques to use on a woman*
- *great techniques to use on a man.*

You can use the techniques in this chapter as a preliminary to intercourse, during intercourse and to reach orgasm without intercourse.

Some general principles

Great sex requires time. In my focus groups I often ask people what's the maximum they've spent in bed for sex, and one woman told me 36 hours. Good for her. If you've never spent more than a few minutes over sex then this could be the biggest thing to happen to you in your life. Great sex, from start to finish, should always take at least an hour. That's a minimum. A whole afternoon or evening should be devoted to sex now and then – say, once a week. If you can't make this sort of time available for your sex life together then you need to take a long, hard look at your lives and your relationship.

People sometimes ask me: 'But what do you *do* all that time?' Well, that's what this book, but especially this chapter, is all about.

SEX FOR AN HOUR

If you've just never thought of spending a long time over sex, if it's always over in a few minutes, then you need some sort of device to help you keep at it for longer. In fact, there is something highly effective and you can usually find it in every bedroom. It's called a clock.

Now I know that people often condemn 'sex by numbers' but numbers can be useful at times. The number 'one', for a start. The idea is very simply that you and your partner will have sex for *one hour*. This can include sexual intercourse but is not exclusively confined to intercourse. Most men like the idea, yet find it difficult to delay ejaculating for so long. Quite a lot of women, on the other hand, are resistant to the idea of hour-long sex on the grounds that it will make them sore and become uncomfortable, repetitive and just plain boring. Part of the exercise is to make sure that it isn't any of those things.

The best way to go about this is to place a large (and stern-looking) clock where you can easily see it, and to pace yourselves accordingly. (Some lubricant close to hand will be a good idea, too.) It's amazing how men who normally ejaculate quite quickly find that the discipline of the clock keeps things under control. The notion of simply 'going on as long as possible' is too vague for most men; the specific goal of one hour, on the other hand, is the sort of target that men find a challenge.

Run through all the techniques in this chapter. If both of you agree, you could also set a goal for intercourse alone of, say, 15 minutes or 20 minutes within that hour, or whatever is significantly longer than you've managed before. Keep an eye on the clock and see how things go.

Of course, it's preferable that both of you know about and agree with sex by the clock. If you've made up your mind to try for an hour without telling your partner, you'll have to use plenty of cues ('Don't orgasm yet, I'm enjoying it so much.').

Naturally, you won't always use a clock. This is just a way of helping you to develop a feel for longer sex sessions. Once you've achieved that, you can put the clock away.

Great warm-up techniques to use on yourself

I'm assuming that you've set the scene as described in the previous chapter. You've kissed, you've cuddled, you've put on some music, you've adjusted the lights, the room is filled with perfume, you're taking a shower together and you're ready to have great sex.

The next thing you might like to do is masturbate. Yes, masturbate. There are several ways in which masturbation leads to great sex. It isn't something you only do when you're alone. In the first place, it's essential to see how your partner masturbates, because it's the quickest and best way of learning how he or she likes to be touched. Second, watching your partner masturbate is exciting (although probably more so for men than for women). Third, the sensation of masturbating together is quite different to either solo masturbation or intercourse. Try lying side by side and masturbating. It's like a journey to the stars in separate rockets but flying in formation. And, finally, masturbation is a way of preparing your body.

Obviously, your partner can also do things to 'get you going', but the freedom to masturbate in your partner's presence is a sort of 'insurance policy'. A woman might like to play a vibrator on her clitoris, for example. Meanwhile, a man might like to be paying attention to his prostate gland, as described in Chapter 3.

If you're working your way towards intercourse, a man probably won't actually want to ejaculate at this point, but a woman can enjoy one or more orgasms by masturbation. One wonderful style is for the man to be a human armchair (see Chapter 4) and hold his partner while she plays with herself. He can put his hand on top of hers or she can take his hand and use it to pleasure herself. A lot of men find it very exciting and intimate to be holding their lovers when they orgasm.

Another style is to sit facing one another, legs apart. This way you can see one another's genitals and facial expressions and, if you wish, look into one another's eyes for a more intimate feeling.

In fact, there are all kinds of possibilities. There's no reason why you shouldn't adopt any posture that appeals to you. Be uninhibited. Use everything you would when you're on your own.

Unisex techniques

Here are some techniques that both of you can use during your hour of sex. Techniques to be used specifically on a woman or specifically on a man are given after this section.

Nowhere on the male or female body is so responsive that you can just 'grab' it before there's been any arousal. In fact, certain parts of the body can feel so unresponsive at first that you just give up on them. However, once an area is flooded with blood it becomes significantly more sensitive. You'll be amazed at the difference if you just allow time to take care of things.

ULTIMATE KISSING

Make your kisses even more intimate by taking a mouthful of something pleasant and 'kissing' it into your partner's mouth. It works best with drinks but it can also be good with some foods (for example, nuts). But the most powerful thing you can do is take turns at biting and sucking one another's tongues, either as foreplay or during intercourse. The sensations will go straight to your genitals.

LUBRICATE YOUR BODIES

Everything feels much more sensitive when it's slippery. So why not lubricate *all* of your bodies for the ultimate skin experience? An excellent technique (see 'Massage' in Chapter 4, page 77) is for just one of you to apply a liberal quantity of something suitable to your own body and then to rub yourself all over your partner. Don't forget to do it on both sides. Body oil is probably the best but sun lotion works too, and you can always raid the kitchen – use lighter oils such as grapeseed and olive oil. Don't put any lubricant on the genitals until you've finished oral sex (unless you're certain you don't mind the taste) and don't get any oil on condoms (it can make holes in them) or inside the vagina (it can cause infections).

HAND RIDING

One of you caresses yourself in the way you like. The other places his or her hand on your hand and 'rides' it. In this way your partner can learn exactly where and how you like to be touched. Once you've done that, try reversing hands. In other words, the person who is going to be caressed takes hold of his or her partner's hand and moves it around.

PUBIC HAIR TWEAK

The more blood you can get into the pelvic area, the more sensitive and responsive it will become. Take a group of your partner's pubic hairs between finger and thumb and tug them sharply. Then another group. Then another. Check that it's having the right effect – neither too weak nor too painful. Then do it a few more times. Also give your partner a few sharp slaps on the buttocks, if he or she likes it (a little bit of fantasy complements this very well). See Chapters 7 and 9 for more on these subjects.

THE BIG TOE

With the nail closely trimmed, the big toe can be a very effective sex toy. Try masturbating, facing one another, each with one leg between your partner's legs. A man can use his big toe on his partner's vulva and she can use her big toe on his anus.

IMSAK

According to legend, a man could satisfy a dozen of his harem in one night using *imsak*, an Arab word signifying 'retention'.

But, in fact, there's no reason a woman can't equally initiate *imsak*, especially if she's on top, so I'm considering it here as a unisex system. On the surface, *imsak* is fairly straightforward but it requires a high degree of control on the part of the man. The idea is that you repeatedly build excitement then separate for a minute or two to cool off. Skilled lovers might have ten or more bouts over the space of, say, an hour. There are two advantages to *imsak* for a modern couple. The first is that it prolongs the whole wonderful experience of sex. The second is that, if the man decides to ejaculate at the end, he will experience the most explosive and extended sensations, due to the relentless build-up of sexual fluids. The woman will also enjoy extended orgasm, but only if she hasn't had previous orgasms. Because of its ability to maintain an altered state of consciousness for long periods, *imsak* can be used in tantric sex (see below).

Insight

In between bouts, you can carry on kissing, cuddling and caressing, or even share food and wine. But don't let things cool down too far because repeated entry into a less-excited vagina can cause feelings of soreness rather than pleasure. Some older men may have a problem regaining full erection after a few breaks. The secret is to keep relaxed and self-stimulate as necessary.

TANTRIC SEX

There are lots of misconceptions about tantric sex, largely because a number of self-proclaimed Western 'gurus' have been giving courses and writing books about things that have little or nothing to do with the authentic traditions. What defines tantric sex is that it's sex for spiritual purposes. Having said that, it's true that spiritual experiences are far more likely to come during the extended sessions that are possible when both partners experience multiple orgasms. I'll have more to say about multiple orgasms and tantric sex in Chapters 7 and 8, but if you're really interested in the subject you might also like to read *Get Intimate with Tantric Sex*.

Great techniques to use on a woman

In Chapter 2 you learned about a woman's sexual apparatus. Now we're going to find out what to do with it.

If you are a woman, don't be in the least bit embarrassed to ask your partner to spend longer over the things that give you pleasure. In my focus groups, men tell me how proud and satisfied they feel when they give their partners gratification not only with their penises but also with their fingers and tongues. *The Hite Report on Male Sexuality* (Shere Hite, 1981) found exactly the same. Men spoke of being 'thrilled' and of feeling 'wild' when their partners had orgasms when they themselves did not. Most likely your partner will be very happy if you ask for more because it confirms that you enjoy what he does.

SKIN

The neck and the ears are good places to start. After that, move on to the rest of the skin. The general principle is to begin gently and to gradually increase intensity. In other words, start with breathing on the skin, tickling, caressing, kissing and sucking and move on to scratching, pinching and slapping. Obviously, you don't want to actually hurt your partner so check that what you're doing isn't too hard. Blood will surge into the area you're working on, turning the skin pink and increasing sensitivity. The more widespread your activities, the more likely your partner is to experience a whole body orgasm in due course, but there will obviously come a point when you concentrate on the inner thighs and buttocks. Now and then, spanking can be fun (see Chapter 9).

You can add interest by smearing your partner with something tasty and licking it off. Things like chocolate spread, honey, yoghurt, whipped cream and mayonnaise are all good, depending on your taste. But keep food away from the vulva and vagina as it can encourage infections.

BREASTS AND NIPPLES

Try circling your partner's breasts very delicately with the tip of a finger, gradually working your way in to the areolas and nipples. Try licking and sucking. Use your teeth only very delicately. Men's nipples aren't very elastic but a woman's nipples can be drawn out as much as 2.5 cm (1 inch). Ask your partner which part of which breast feels the most pleasurable (because the two breasts may not be the same) and concentrate there. Everyone assumes it must be the nipple, but that isn't necessarily the case. Only a tiny percentage of women orgasm from breast stimulation. On the other hand, when you're stimulating your partner's genitals, she'll almost certainly find that breast stimulation intensifies the excitement even more.

THE VULVA (INCLUDING THE CLITORIS)

Assuming your partner isn't yet completely naked, you could start by caressing her vulva and particularly her clitoris through her underwear. If she's very sensitive, she may enjoy this diffused sensation more than direct contact.

Insight

Place your knee between your lover's thighs while you're kissing her lips or nibbling her nipples. She can rub her vulva against it and give herself some very nice sensations.

Once your partner is naked, however, your lips and tongue are good tools with which to get things going. They're soft and plump and also wet, so if your partner hasn't produced much lubrication your saliva will help. While you're doing this you'll also become aroused not only by the view but also by her natural perfume. If she's removed the hair from her outer labia you'll both respond all the quicker.

You can give your partner oral stimulation (cunnilingus) in various positions. The most comfortable for her is probably lying on her back with her legs apart. A pillow under her buttocks will make everything more accessible. She could also raise her hips up by bending her knees, putting her feet flat on the bed and pushing up. It's not a comfortable position but it's an excitingly tense one. Another way to create tension is for her to kneel with her thighs apart and lean back on her arms or against some pillows. Other possibilities include the woman on her hands and knees or standing. For simultaneous oral sex, in the '69' position, see the section on men below.

If you don't know, ask your partner what she likes. As a general principle, start by licking the entire area – her labia, the entrance to her vagina and the clitoral hood and stem. As she becomes aroused, the outer lips will pull back and the inner lips enlarge. Now you can lick each of the inner lips in turn and play with them between *your* lips. Then concentrate a little more on the clitoris. Try strokes of your tongue to the sides, and then the hood, and, if she's not too sensitive, the clitoris itself. Try slow strokes and fast strokes. Take the clitoris gently between your lips and play with it. You can also try humming – the vibrations can be quite thrilling. Alternate with long licks from her anus up to her mons area. When she's really turned on, she'll press against you. Just put your tongue out and down as far as it will go and let her grind her clitoris against it, or try jabbing it against the entrance. If you have a tongue that extends a long way, insert it into her vagina.

A word of warning: On no account blow into the vagina. It will do nothing for your partner's pleasure and, in certain circumstances, it could actually kill her.

> ### Insight
> Take a small mouthful of wine, let it warm, then dribble it onto your partner's vulva. Provided it's a wine with a low alcoholic content, it will give her an interesting tingle.
> **A word of caution:** Avoid strong wine (over 12 per cent) and certainly don't use spirits because they will *hurt*.

When you want to use your mouth and tongue to arouse your partner somewhere else, you can continue the stimulation of the vulva with your fingers. This could be a good moment to introduce some additional lubrication, either saliva or something from a sex shop (see Chapter 9). Some women don't like being kissed after their partners have performed oral sex on them, which is a shame because it means the kissing is over. If your partner feels that way, see if she can't overcome her squeamishness. It's no different to her licking her own fingers as she plays with herself.

When you're using your fingers (say two, or your thumb alone), gradually increase the pace. As your partner approaches orgasm, you'll have to move about as fast as you can manage. But when she actually does start having her orgasm she'll almost certainly prefer it if you stop all movement and just press. Most women don't like to be touched for a few seconds after the orgasm is over because the clitoris is then highly sensitive (just as the penis can be). Similarly, the area can become quite numb after a lot of attention. Obviously, communication is the key to getting it right since every woman is different.

Insight

There are ways of intensifying the sensations. One is to gently spread her inner lips while you work on her clitoris. Another is to put the palm of your free hand on her mons and gently pull the skin up towards her navel. Both of these techniques will expose the glans of the clitoris (see Chapter 2) for a more powerful stimulus. But don't overdo it. Incidentally, some women enjoy very nice sensations simply by having their mons areas rotated by their partners. Gently slapping the vulva a few times can increase the blood flow.

THE VAGINA AND G-SPOT

The vagina is not generally the place to begin. If you're both feeling hot there's no reason you can't go straight for a quickie, but that's not great sex. For great sex you should already have done the things described earlier in this chapter and the previous chapter and only then should you start on your partner's vagina by inserting one well-lubricated finger. Gradually, explore further inside. Locate the G-spot as described in Chapter 2. Now gently massage it. Try different kinds of strokes to see what feels best to her. Press different places. Round and round. From side to side. And the 'come here' movement with the pad of the forefinger. Next try two well-lubricated fingers and see what happens when you gently knead the G-spot between them. If your partner has been practising as recommended earlier in the book, she'll be able to guide you. If you're doing it right, you should be able to feel the G-spot swelling up. If you want to try for a G-spot ejaculation right now, read the relevant section again in Chapter 2.

By sliding your fingers in and out, you may be able to bring your partner to orgasm. More likely, you'll have to stimulate her clitoris simultaneously, either with your other hand or with your tongue.

Insight

Switching stimulation backwards and forwards between the clitoris and the G-spot is a great way of extending her orgasms. When she feels almost ready to come from clitoral stimulation change to the G-spot, and when she feels almost ready to come from that, switch back to the clitoris. And so on. With good communication it should be possible to maintain a state of pre-orgasmic bliss and the eventual orgasm should be longer than usual and quite shattering.

GREAT WAYS OF MOVING

The universal image of intercourse is of the man thrusting in and out while the woman lies still. In fact, either or both of you can move (depending on position), and in various different ways.

Here are some things that a man can do with his penis during intercourse.

▶ *Try using the penis like a finger rather than a piston. Explore the vulva, including the clitoris, then inside the vagina – the entrance, the roof (especially the G-spot), the floor, the sides and the cervix (at the far end).*

▶ *Try different combinations of deep and shallow penetration. For example, nine shallow and one deep, or five shallow and one deep, or one shallow and one deep.*

▶ *Hold your penis in your fist with about half its length protruding. Like this you can circle the glans within the entrance or apply pressure to a particular point, making it a great technique for stimulating the G-spot. Your hand will also automatically stimulate her clitoris. You can enhance this effect by placing your thumb so that it presses against the clitoris with each thrust.*

▶ *Rather than moving in and out, make the penis 'wave' inside the vagina by changing the angle of your hips. In the missionary position you can achieve the same effect by leaning further forwards then back. As you lean forwards so you make contact with the clitoris.*

▶ *Make a 'screwing' movement by rotating your hips. This is particularly effective in some of the rear-entry positions.*

▶ *With the penis inserted to the maximum and without moving it within the vagina, simply grind your pelvic area against your partner. You'll receive almost no stimulation but she'll feel quite a bit, making this a useful technique for prolonging intercourse.*

▶ *One of the most exciting moments for a woman is the feeling of the labia and entrance to the vagina being opened. So, guys, don't just do it once. Do it 10, 50 or 100 times. Withdraw completely, then, after a moment, slide back in. See what happens when you vary the length of time between penetrations. One second, five seconds, ten seconds...*

Insight

I've already mentioned a clock as a way of learning to pace yourselves. It can also be useful as a sort of training aid for a man during intercourse. It doesn't work for all men, but in my focus groups a significant proportion did find that it helped them. If you've never been able to continue for longer than, say, five minutes then set yourself a target of ten minutes.

(Contd)

Be determined not to orgasm until the ten minutes is up.
If you achieve that, then extend the time again in your next
session. By giving a specific target to aim for, many men find
that they achieve better control. Naturally, you won't always
make love by the clock, it's just to help you learn.

ANAL SEX

Done well, and only if it's done well, anal sex can add a very
special extra dimension to lovemaking. In her memoir *The
Surrender*, mentioned in Chapter 2 (see 'Taking it further'), Toni
Bentley describes it as an experience of eternity and even of God.
How can this be? In fact, this whole area is packed with nerve
endings and, among others, is served by the pudendal nerve, which
also connects to the clitoris and vagina. Another source of pleasure
may be a mysterious structure known as the coccygeal body,
which is located between the rectum and the tailbone. In Tantra,
this is known as the 'Kundalini gland' and is seen as the seat of
a special energy. True or not, quite a lot of women rate the anus
equal to the vagina in terms of sensation. But it's the psychology
of anal intercourse that's so different. To a woman it can feel like
the ultimate demonstration of her willingness to open herself up
to her lover (and, for those of a mystical inclination, to the whole
universe).

Is anal sex 'unnatural'? Well, in surveys, between a quarter and a
third of couples seem to have tried it, although the proportion that
practises it regularly is much lower. In any event, what's 'natural'
or 'unnatural' has no relevance. Human beings have long done
things that aren't 'natural' and that's what defines us as a species.
If you both enjoy it, that's all that counts.

Insight

Anal sex can pose a health risk. There are bacteria happily
established in the anal canal and rectum that could cause
serious infections if they get into the vagina or urethra. For
that reason, anything that's been inside the anal canal/rectum
(finger, sex toy, etc.) must be thoroughly washed before

anything else is done with it. To avoid accidental infection, it's a good idea for a man to designate one hand as his 'anal hand'. In addition to the normal bacteria, there are additional hazards connected with diseases and viruses such as hepatitis and HIV. Therefore, only indulge in anal play in the context of a long-term relationship in which you're completely confident there's no possibility of spreading illness. Also remember that the anal canal and rectum are very delicate and have no natural lubrication. If you don't have a suitable artificial lubricant then *do not* indulge in anal sex.

First of all, a little biology lesson. The most important point to understand is that, because of the cunning way the digestive system functions, the parts of the digestive tract concerned with anal sex are clear of waste matter for long periods. Those parts are the anus, the anal canal and the rectum. The place that waste is actually stored is even further inside the body, in the colon. It's only when the colon moves the waste out of storage that it finds its way into the rectum and, if you're paying attention, you'll be able to feel the muscular contractions that do it. At that point, you'll probably experience a sensation of fullness and pressure. If you then go to the toilet your rectum will be empty until the colon's next contractions, which might not be for several hours. So the first rule of anal penetration is timing. If a woman has recently emptied the 'short-term holding area' that is the rectum, then she has the 'green light' for anal sex. If not, then she'll probably want to defer anal penetration until another session.

The first stage in anal play is stimulation of the anus itself, that's to say, the visible sphincter or ring of muscle. While having sex in the Cuddly bears position (see Chapter 6) try running a *lubricated* finger along the groove of your partner's buttocks and then circling her anus. If she enjoys that, and only if she does, try pushing your forefinger (nail well-trimmed) in just a little way. The anus is under conscious control, so if your finger goes in easily it means your partner is relaxed and enjoying the sensations. If it's difficult to enter it means she's tense. In that case, try a little more circling. That's enough for the first session.

The next stage, another time, is to play with her anal canal. That's the smooth tube of 2.5 cm to 5 cm (1–2 inches) between the external sphincter and the internal sphincter, which, being governed by the autonomic nervous system, is *not* under conscious control. There should never be any waste matter in this area and therefore no cause for embarrassment. Once again, have sex in the Cuddly bears position and then, using masses of lubricant and after 'warming up' her anus, gently push a finger (nail trimmed short) a little way inside. *Do not* then begin thrusting in and out. More enjoyable are simply the sensations of penetration, of being opened, and of the very smooth surface of the canal being sensitively stimulated. Very gently explore different movements and ask your partner what feels nicest. At first she may not know herself because the sensations will feel quite strange, but slowly turning the finger is usually good. Have several sessions like this until your partner feels completely comfortable and happy to accept a thumb and then two or three fingers. With a forefinger in her anus you could also try putting the forefinger of your other hand into her vagina and gently squeezing the perineal sponge between the two. Some couples go no further than this with anal play.

Insight

When you put your finger into your partner's anal canal you'll be able to feel your penis inside her vagina. That can be very exciting for you. And because your finger will be pressing her vaginal wall into closer contact with your penis, that will provide additional excitement for her. You could also slip an anal vibrator into her (see Chapter 9). Both of you will be able to feel that.

It may be, however, that during a sex session you both feel you'd like to go 'all the way'. In that case, as foreplay, repeat stages one and two. Once she's ready, gently push your forefinger against the internal sphincter. Remember this sphincter is *not* under conscious control but the more relaxed she feels generally, the easier it will be. Don't force it. If that's a success, continue the anal sex play unhurriedly until her anus is so relaxed that it remains slightly open on its own. That's the time to try entry with your penis.

Don't forget to use liberal amounts of lubricant. Initially, leave the head of your penis inside the anal canal. Don't go further until she's ready and then only very slowly.

Insight

A man will need a much stronger erection to get into the anal canal than into the vagina. A woman can help by reaching behind with both hands (her head resting on a pillow) and spreading her buttocks apart. Another trick is for her to reach back between her legs and insert her own forefinger into her anal canal. The man then holds his penis above her finger and uses it to 'shoehorn' himself inside, without the possibility of skidding into the vagina. There are special sex toys for the anus that can be used to relax the sphincters (see Chapter 9).

What next? It's probably best to leave that to her. Let her explore her own sensations by taking control of movements. If she begins pushing backwards against you (in the Cuddly bears position) then you'll know she wants to go deeper. Should you ejaculate? If you're wearing a condom (see below) you could, although she'd probably prefer ejaculation in the vagina, but I'd recommend not ejaculating otherwise. That would be messy and the semen may well irritate the anal canal and rectum, and the health risk increases, too. On the other hand, *she* can certainly come – reach around to her clitoris and caress it.

You'll probably now want to finish off with vaginal intercourse, which means you'll have to go and wash first. She may also want to wash. It's a good idea. Doesn't that destroy the atmosphere? Not at all. Just look upon it as *imsak*, as described above. Or view it like an interval in the theatre, so that when you return to your places you're looking forward to the next Act. Or you could wash together in the shower and resume lovemaking there.

Caution: In porn videos you may see a man transfer his penis from his partner's anus to her vagina, or her mouth. Never, ever copy that. It's highly dangerous.

I'll now deal with the question of condoms and latex gloves. In my opinion you shouldn't have anal sex *at all* if there's any risk of spreading infection. If you're completely confident on that point then condoms and gloves are a barrier to the kind of intimacy that is one of the aims of anal sex. However, if condoms are your chosen contraceptive then there's a strong argument for wearing one during anal sex, firstly because there's always the possibility of sliding into the vagina rather than the anus and, secondly, because semen could just about migrate from the anal area into the vagina. If you're using sex toys (see Chapter 9) you can also use condoms to cover them. You can then transfer a vibrator that's been in the anal canal/rectum to the vagina by removing the old condom and putting a fresh one on. Cleaning the toys afterwards is also much easier.

How often should you incorporate anal penetration into your lovemaking? That, of course, is for you and your partner to decide together. But bear in mind that if you reserve anal sex for 'special' occasions, such as your birthday, your partner's body will never get used to it and she'll probably never enjoy it. So it's worth trying to agree that you'll give anal intercourse, say, six goes during the course of a month. Then decide how you both feel about it.

Insight

In my focus groups, women ask me why men like anal sex. There are probably several reasons. Experimentation, the thrill of the 'forbidden', the resistance of the anal sphincter which gives men that sense of domination and triumph, a tight barrel and, paradoxically perhaps, a lack of stimulation (because the rectum doesn't do anything), which allows a man to continue for a long time. Yet I suspect the biggest reason why men like it is because of the feeling that a woman has given everything with no holding back. And those women who like it also like it for the same reason – as the ultimate act of opening up to someone they love.

THE FULL SYMPHONY

During an extended session you might receive fellatio (see below) and then penetrate your partner's vagina, and then her anus, and then (after washing) her vagina again. From the woman's point of view (assuming she likes all three) this variety helps prevent her becoming numb from too much concentration on the vulva/vagina.

Insight

Anal penetration adds an extra dimension to sex but it's not one that all women want to explore. If you're a woman whose partner is eager to experiment but you're not, what should you do? Of course, you must say how you feel. Point out all the lovely things you *can* do together and suggest you both concentrate on making the most of those.

Great techniques to use on a man

In the bad old days, women tended to be passive in sex. Thankfully, that's no longer the case, because both men and women enjoy sex more when women are active. In Chapter 2 you learned about a man's sexual apparatus. Now we're going to find out what to do with it.

SKIN, BREASTS, NIPPLES

Men are far more genitally focused than women. It's how their brains are wired up. It can be fun to try to 'unwire' them by putting some effort into all the other bits, and over time it can work. For example, if you stimulate a man's nipples while also stimulating his penis you may be able to 'train' the nipples to become more responsive. The same goes for kissing and blowing in ears. Generally, the same suggestions that were made for women apply to men but less so.

THE PENIS

Most men love fellatio (oral sex), or a 'blow job'. One way of going about it is the well-known '69' position. While he's busy with his mouth on your clitoris and vulva, you can be applying your lips and tongue to his penis. Take control by keeping your hand around the base of the penis. The 69 can be lying side by side, or you can be on top, or he can be on top. But there is a problem with 69. Your tongue, which is your most effective weapon, will be on the 'wrong' side of his glans. For the most electric effect, it needs to be applied to the underside (frenulum side).

Is there a better way? An excellent position is one that he hopefully uses on you. That is, he lies on his back with his legs apart and you lie between them. Like this, you're both comfortable and you can see by his facial expressions the kind of effect you're having. If he wants more tension, he can raise himself up by bending his knees with his feet flat on the bed and pushing with his arms. Alternatively, he can kneel with legs apart, then lean back on his arms or against some cushions.

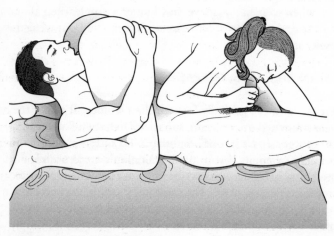

Figure 5.1 Cunnilingus and fellatio in the '69' position.

Yet another possibility is that you lie on your back with your head on a pillow and he straddles your chest. While you're busy with his penis he can reach behind to work on your clitoris with his fingers or a vibrator.

Insight

You can produce some very interesting effects by drinking something just before performing fellatio. For example, swallowing a mouthful of tea will produce a lovely warm sensation. Then you could switch to something cold from the fridge. Similarly, you could put a 'dressing' on his penis then lick it off – try yoghurt, whipped cream or jam. (If you're going to have intercourse afterwards, it's best to wash foodstuffs off, otherwise they may encourage vaginal infections.)

Some men like to ejaculate in their lovers' mouths. Some women are excited by this, some don't mind, and some hate the idea. Semen actually has very little taste and certainly isn't harmful. A major objection is that a man who has had an orgasm this way won't be able to pleasure you with intercourse until his refractory period has passed. In rare cases, that could be a few minutes. More commonly it could be 30 minutes or so, and if your lover is a mature man, you might have to wait until tomorrow.

Of course, you can use your mouth without actually taking his penis inside. You can simply lick him with your tongue as if he's an ice cream. In fact, why not put some real ice cream on him? Apart from the underside of the glans, the underside of the shaft, along that dark line, is another good place.

There's also a variety of things that you can do with your fingers. Don't forget to use lots of lubrication. If you use anything other than saliva then it's best to do the fellatio first and use your fingers afterwards, otherwise you'll be tasting whatever lubricant you've used.

If your partner doesn't yet have a very strong erection, simply place a finger and thumb opposite one another on the outside of the foreskin (assuming he has one) and then use the foreskin to massage the glans. Once he's erect, the foreskin will be stretched and more or less disappear. You'll now be able to rub the underside of the glans directly, including the frenulum itself. Also run a finger or two up and down the dark line on the underside of the penis. Now make your hand into a sort of vagina and, adding fresh lubrication if necessary, run it up and down the penis from top to bottom. Also try turning your closed hand around the penis, as if turning a round doorknob (but don't turn his penis). Lastly, run your closed hand once again down the shaft, but this time holding tightly enough to take any loose skin with you. When you reach the bottom of the shaft, keep it there and, with your other hand, touch the taut skin as well as the glans.

If you go on to have intercourse, you can use the same technique of holding the skin taut; this is known as '*à la florentine*'. Here are some other ideas to try during intercourse:

▸ *Take hold of the base of your partner's penis in your fist and experiment with different ways of moving it. Try rubbing the glans against your clitoris or circling it inside the entrance to your vagina. In one of the woman-on-top-positions you can also move up and down on it, letting your clitoris bump against your hand.*

▸ *In one of the woman-on-top-positions, try sliding up and down the full length of the penis. Try short movements. Try withdrawing from the penis completely and then just sinking down enough to tantalize your lips.*

▸ *In one of the woman-on-top-positions, try leaning forward and back, thus changing the angle of the penis inside you.*

▸ *In a rear-entry position, ask your man to stay still while you take control. Experiment with short and long movements.*

▸ *Try rotating your hips in a churning motion.*

▸ *Open two fingers into an upside down V, put them either side of your vulva and use them to apply extra stimulation to your man's penis. (At the same time your thumb can be working on your clitoris.)*

▸ *Try inserting one or more fingers into your vagina along with the penis – you'll find there's room.*

▶ *Try inserting a finger into your anal canal/rectum so that you can feel his penis inside you and, at the same time, apply extra pressure to it.*

▶ *On each out-stroke that your man makes, squeeze your PC muscle. He'll feel your vagina tighten around him, giving him the most marvellous massage each time he withdraws.*

Insight

The technique of squeezing the penis with the vaginal muscles is known as *kabazzah* or *pompoir*. Women who practise the art can almost hold the penis inside the vagina and stroke it from one end to the other, so that the man has no need to move. For that, the PC muscles need to be exceptionally strong (see Chapter 11).

THE PERINEUM AND SCROTUM

Normally the scrotum and the perineum (the area between the anus and the testicles) aren't very sensitive but once a man is aroused they become so. During intercourse, tip a generous dollop of lubricant onto your hand and then caress him there. He'll love it even more if he's shaved – something you could do for him as a little bit of foreplay.

THE ANUS AND PROSTATE

Earlier in the chapter I wrote about anal sex for women. Hopefully you've been experimenting with it and found some techniques that give you pleasure. If anything, a man's pleasure is even greater. But if your man has never tried any kind of anal sex you may have a psychological barrier to overcome first. You see, some heterosexual men are afraid that the enjoyment of anal stimulation must mean they have homosexual tendencies. So you may have to reassure your man that that's complete rubbish. Quite simply the anus and anal canal are packed with nerve endings, which can generate some exquisite sensations, regardless of sexual orientation. Your man might also bristle at the idea of taking the 'passive' role of being penetrated, rather then being the one doing the penetrating. But if you can persuade him then he's in for a great time.

The best way to start is by caressing his scrotum and perineum during intercourse, as described above. Don't forget the lubricant because it makes an enormous difference. Let a finger stray onto his anal area. If he likes it, go a little bit further by circling his anus. And if he likes that, then push your fingertip inside. You should be able to do this fairly easily in one of the side-by-side positions or in one of the missionary-type positions, especially if he's squatting between your thighs (see Chapter 6). Unless he has some psychological hang-ups about anal penetration I guarantee this will drive him wild and you should feel him stiffen inside you. In fact, it's such a powerful technique that if he's close to ejaculation this alone may be enough to push him over.

Once he's comfortable with the whole idea you can also combine anal play with fellatio. Or he could lie on his back while you masturbate him with one hand and penetrate him with the other. Or he could kneel with his face resting on a pillow while you pleasure him from behind. Keep in mind that, as with you, anal play isn't anywhere near as powerful on its own. Its main function is to reinforce arousal. So keep up the stimulation of his penis.

Insight

The nerves that govern the anus respond most strongly to the sensation of opening. So rather than thrust your finger in and out, increase stimulation by increasing the number of fingers, one at a time (all with short nails). If you have small hands you should easily be able to get four fingertips into the anal canal. Then, gently, try rotating them. Don't forget the lubrication, because the anal canal has none of its own.

What about going deeper? Basically, the anatomy and the methods described in 'Great techniques to use on a woman' (see page 94) also apply to a man. So you need to know if it's a good time or not. In other words, is there any waste matter in his rectum? He should know.

Men have one more reason than women to enjoy deep anal penetration. That's because the male prostate is located against the wall of the rectum about 5.5 cm (2.25 inches) in from the anus (whereas a woman's is stimulated via the vagina). As we saw in Chapter 3, stimulation of the prostate increases the output of prostatic fluid, making ejaculations longer and more powerful. Quite a lot of men also find the whole thing very pleasurable in itself.

If you're not sure how to find the prostate with your finger refer to Chapter 3. You can stimulate it during intercourse or while masturbating him or while he masturbates himself. If you're not keen on using your finger, a properly designed sex toy should find the prostate all by itself and you can even leave it in place throughout sex.

Insight

Not all men derive enjoyable sensations from prostate massage. In fact, the older the man, the less likely it is. Even so, the opening of the anus and the penetration of the rectum will still be enormously stimulating to the prostate, both increasing excitement and the length and power of ejaculation. Note, however, that overemphasis on anal play can have the opposite of the desired effect on the penis, causing it to subside. So for an older man the rule is, do it but don't overdo it.

Simultaneous orgasms

Simultaneous orgasm is certainly one of the greatest experiences in sex. To enjoy the orgasm at the same time is both exciting and uniting, and it brings the active part of the session to a natural end.

If the woman has orgasms first, that's no problem. On the contrary, in a great sex session she should have several before her partner. But she can still have one final one – probably a 'bigger' one – at the same time as the man. And she should. The real problem is if the man ejaculates before his partner has had even one orgasm. Unless he's unusually virile, his erection will subside and the only way he can then continue to excite his partner is by using his tongue and fingers or a vibrator. Unfortunately, quite frankly, his heart won't be in it any longer because he'll already be succumbing to the hormones that make him feel unexcited and even sleepy.

If you want to co-ordinate final orgasms – and I recommend that you do – you need to discover ways of unleashing your orgasm and your partner's more or less at will. It helps a lot if the woman orgasms easily and the man has good control. If that isn't your case, take a look at Chapter 8.

First, agree that you *will* aim for simultaneous orgasms. Don't just leave it as a vague hope. You're going to have to co-operate and that requires a sort of plan that you will both follow.

Second, practise the techniques that are most likely to tip your partner over into orgasm. In other words, when you feel your own orgasm building, you need to be able to do something to your partner that will make him or her orgasm as well. Something powerful. Unfortunately, there's no technique that will make a man or woman orgasm in a few seconds starting from zero. However, there are techniques that will make most men and women orgasm very rapidly if they're already highly excited:

▶ *The most effective physical thing that a woman can do to a man is to push a finger into his anus (his anal area already having been made excited and lubricated).*
▶ *The most effective physical thing a man can do to a woman is to let her masturbate herself.*

There are men who don't want their partners to masturbate during intercourse. It makes them feel failures. If your man thinks you should only orgasm as a result of what he's doing, this attitude needs straightening out right away.

I've already written about the importance of being able to masturbate together. If you haven't done so already, let him watch you masturbate. Once he's enjoyed that (which he will), you're on your way to introducing masturbation into intercourse. Always do it in a positive way, and remember, never criticize failure but always praise success. Explain that you are the only one who can manipulate your clitoris in order to orgasm at precisely the right moment.

Communication plays a big part in success. You have to make it clear to your partner that your own orgasm is building. You can simply say so, of course. That's a good start. But it will be much more effective if you communicate your excitement at the same time. Excitement is, well, exciting. It's catching. It'll turn your partner on. And talk dirty. If necessary, use a fantasy. Use the power of the mind. How? That's the subject of Chapter 7 – but next we'll be turning to great sex positions.

10 THINGS TO REMEMBER

1 *One hour is the minimum for great sex; use a clock to help you until you've learned how to pace things.*

2 *Show one another how you masturbate and enjoy doing it together as a way of building up excitement.*

3 *Stimulate all of the skin surface, paying particular attention to a woman's neck, ears, nipples, areolas and breasts.*

4 *Pay plenty of attention to the clitoris; if you want more clitoral stimulation than your partner is giving, don't be afraid to ask, nor to tell him when your clitoris has had enough.*

5 *Be sure you know how your partner likes her clitoris to be treated, not just up to but also during orgasm.*

6 *If you're massaging the G-spot correctly, you'll feel it swell up.*

7 *The '69' is a well-known position for simultaneous oral sex, but it's not the best position for a man; men like to feel the tongue on the underside of the glans, which means lying between his legs or letting him straddle your chest.*

8 *Keep control of fellatio by holding the base of your partner's penis.*

9 *Both of you should at least try giving and receiving anal stimulation and anal penetration for a few sessions before deciding whether or not to make anal play a regular part of your repertoire.*

10 *The sure keys to simultaneous orgasms are communication, masturbation for her, and anal stimulation for him.*

HOW GREAT IS SEX NOW?

▶ *Have you been able to achieve a sex session of at least an hour?*   Yes/No

▶ *Have you tried masturbating together?*   Yes/No

▶ *Have you run through the repertoire of unisex techniques?*   Yes/No

▶ *Have you given your partner an orgasm from cunnilingus, or have you performed fellatio?*   Yes/No

▶ *Have you told your partner how you like it done?*   Yes/No

▶ *Have you found your partner's G-spot?*   Yes/No

▶ *Have you experimented with different ways of moving during intercourse?*   Yes/No

▶ *Have you explored your partner's anal canal?*   Yes/No

▶ *If 'yes', did your partner enjoy it?*   Yes/No

▶ *Have you explored beyond your partner's anal canal?*   Yes/No

▶ *If 'yes', did your partner enjoy it?*   Yes/No

▶ *Have you been able to create simultaneous orgasms on a regular basis?*   Yes/No

If you answered 'no' to more than three questions, re-read the relevant parts of the chapter and make an effort to put the suggestions into effect. Practising sexual techniques can seem rather cold and unromantic but, as with everything else, it's the way to perfection – or, at least, a much higher standard. Remember that human beings are the only animals to have turned sex into an art form. You'll be using these techniques in conjunction with all the great positions in the next chapter.

6

Great positions

In this chapter you will learn:
- *why you should use lots of different positions*
- *the greatest positions*
- *how to switch positions*
- *positions you can use when comfortable furniture isn't available.*

What's the point of lots of different sex positions? This is a question few people would ever ask. Sex positions, like mountain peaks, are *there*. The more you can bag, and the harder they are, the greater the sense of satisfaction afterwards. On the other hand, some people prefer comfort and, above all, the familiar. In fact, there are excellent reasons for using several different positions.

TEN GREAT REASONS FOR USING DIFFERENT POSITIONS

▶ Different psychology. *In Western culture, whoever is on top tends to have a feeling of 'dominance' while the other tends to feel 'submissive'. In some positions this can be quite extreme. In Eastern culture, on the other hand, the person on top gives energy to the person underneath.*
▶ Different emotion. *There are positions in which you feel very close and intimate, with stimulation all over your bodies. In others, you're connected only at the genitals, isolating and concentrating the impact there.*
▶ Different view. *Some positions provide less visual stimulation; others carry a powerful erotic charge. In some positions, you*

can see how your partner is responding; in others, eyes and faces are hidden from one another.

▶ Different muscular tension. *Some positions create more muscular tension than others. When excitement is boiling up too fast, switch to a position with little tension; when things are going too slowly, switch to a position with high tension, which opens and stretches the thighs, such as the Two triangles (see page 130). The more tension in the body, the more likely you are to experience a whole body orgasm.*

▶ Different stimulation. *Different positions stimulate different areas. For example, rear-entry positions make it easier to stimulate the G-spot with the penis. A man who tends to ejaculate too soon should choose a position that provides less stimulation.*

▶ Variety. *You don't want to make love in the same way every time; introduce novelty.*

▶ Rest. *Sometimes you simply need to rest muscles by switching to a different position.*

▶ Practicality. *When a nice comfortable bed isn't available, you may have to find an unusual solution.*

▶ Entertainment. *Trying different positions is quite simply fun.*

▶ Tackling inhibition. *When you struggle and wriggle and stretch and groan and laugh as you attempt the more outrageous and difficult positions, you'll cast off your inhibitions.*

How many positions are there? One author claims 100, another 365, another 1,000. In reality, there are only a few basic positions but with lots of variations. Even if you just stick to the missionary style, for example, you'll probably still do at least a dozen taking into account all the variations that come more or less naturally.

While you're exploring the positions that follow, here are some of the questions you should ask yourselves:

▶ *How does intercourse feel:*
   (a) *in a position that creates a lot of tension?*
   (b) *in a position that's very relaxed?*
   Which feels best?

▶ *How does intercourse feel:*
   (a) *in a position that allows only shallow penetration?*
   (b) *in a position that permits deep penetration?*
   Which feels best?

▶ *How does intercourse feel:*
   (a) *when you can look into your partner's eyes?*
   (b) *when you can't see your partner's face?*
   Which feels best?

▶ *How does intercourse feel:*
   (a) *in a man-on-top position?*
   (b) *in a woman-on-top position?*
   (c) *with the two of you in roughly equal positions?*
   Which feels best?

▶ *How does intercourse feel:*
   (a) *with natural lubrication alone?*
   (b) *with extra lubrication?*
   Which feels best?

▶ *How does it feel if you resume after separating for:*
   (a) *one second?*
   (b) *10 seconds?*
   (c) *30 seconds?*
   Which feels best?

▶ *How does orgasm feel when:*
   (a) *the penis is at an angle to the vagina?*
   (b) *when the vagina and penis are in perfect alignment?*
   Which feels best?

▶ *How does orgasm feel if:*
   (a) *you both keep moving?*
   (b) *only the man keeps moving?*
   (c) *only the woman keeps moving?*
   (d) *neither of you move?*
   Which feels best?

▶ *How does orgasm feel:*
  (a) *in a 'quickie'?*
  (b) *after a 30-minute session?*
  (c) *after an hour-long session?*
  Which feels best?

---

35 great sex positions...and 32 variations

I asked my focus groups to rate positions on a scale of one to 100 and they're listed here in order of the popularity of the main position (not the variations). There's a space for you and your partner to give your own scores, if you want.

GREAT SEX POSITION NO. 1: THE IMPROVED MISSIONARY POSITION

Everybody knows the Missionary, precisely because it's one of the most natural positions there is. With the woman lying comfortably on her back and the man lying between her open thighs, supporting himself on his hands or elbows, it's intimate, allowing for kissing, talking, eye contact and a range of caresses. The man is slightly but not unduly dominant – which suits the psychology of most couples most of the time. The drawback with the Basic missionary is that movement is restricted.

The improved missionary simply requires the addition of a nice, thick pillow under the woman's buttocks. Not only is her vulva now raised for some intensive cunnilingus, but the man can squat or kneel or arrange himself on one knee with the other leg out behind for a powerful and versatile pattern of thrusting. With the man's weight taken off her, the woman is also more free to move.

Focus group score: 94   Your score: ....

The Improved missionary is a marvellous starting point from which to move seamlessly through a wide variety of variations, mostly with the man squatting or kneeling.

Variation 1. The woman wraps her legs around the man's waist.

Focus group score: 85   Your score: ....

Variation 2. The woman puts one leg on each of the man's shoulders.

Focus group score: 85   Your score: ....

Variation 3. The woman holds her legs wide open and in the air at an angle of about 45 degrees. This sets up tremendous tension.

Focus group score: 85   Your score: ....

Insight

In any position in which either of you have your legs open, up and free (such as variation 3 of the improved missionary) try waggling them vigorously as you approach orgasm. The additional stimulation along your inner thighs and throughout your pelvis will almost certainly send you into delirium.

Variation 4. The woman puts both legs on one of the man's shoulders. (This gives a completely different sensation to variation 2 because the legs are together.)

Focus group score: 83   Your score: ....

Variation 5. The woman wraps her legs around the man's legs.

Focus group score: 81   Your score: ....

Variation 6. The woman closes her legs – some women find they can orgasm more easily with their legs together.

Focus group score: 77   Your score: ....

Variation 7. The woman draws in her legs and crosses them in the famous yoga position known as the 'lotus' (or as close to it as she can manage). This really opens up the vagina but, at the same time, keeps the man from thrusting too deep.

Focus group score: 71   Your score: ....

Variation 8. The woman bends her knees, placing her feet on the man's hips.

Focus group score: 68   Your score: ....

Variation 9. The woman raises her legs and clamps them against his hips.

Focus group score: 63   Your score: ....

Variation 10. The man (sitting back on his feet) pulls the woman's hips up onto his thighs and she helps support herself with her feet on the bed, beside his feet.

Focus group score: 56   Your score: ....

Variation 11. The woman lifts her hips and arches her back with her feet on the bed (also a sexy position in which to perform cunnilingus on her). The position known in yoga as the 'bridge' is an extreme version in which the woman dramatically arches her back and lifts her pelvis high. The higher the bridge, the greater the tension.

Focus group score: 52   Your score: ....

Variation 12. The man turns right around (like a propeller) without withdrawing his penis (fun to try but not actually very exciting).

Focus group score: 38   Your score: ....

GREAT SEX POSITION NO. 2: THE BALL

This is really a variation on the Improved missionary but it's such a wonderful position it deserves a name of its own. I call it the Ball because the woman feels a little like a ball and you both have a ball. The woman draws her knees back towards her breasts and, with her legs well bent, places her feet on her lover's shoulders.

Focus group score: 91   Your score: ....

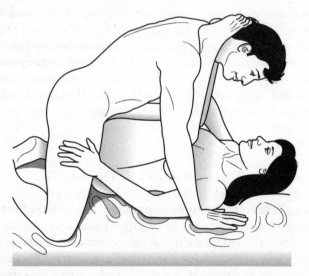

Figure 6.1 The Ball.

GREAT SEX POSITION NO. 3: THE EXHIBITIONIST

This, too, is a variation on the Improved missionary and, in fact, a more extreme version of the Ball. The woman swings her open legs back over her head, as if she was going to do a backwards head-over-heels. She can place her arms behind her knees or even, if she's supple enough, hold her ankles with her hands. The man can help by *gently* nudging her back with his body and by pushing against the underside of her thighs with his arms.

He can follow the movement by rising into a squatting position, or squatting on one leg with the other out behind. In rolling backwards from the Improved missionary, the woman gives the man an exciting – and dominating – view of her genitals, and enjoys the *frisson* of exhibitionism.

Focus group score: 89   Your score: ....

GREAT SEX POSITION NO. 4: GOODBYE WORLD

This is yet another derivative of the Improved missionary but, again, the sensations are sufficiently different for it to merit its own name. The man, from a kneeling position, leans forward to put his arms right around his partner's back. She puts not just her arms but also her legs around his back. This is a tremendously close position, with heads touching side by side. You can co-ordinate breathing and whisper in one another's ears. The world no longer exists. There are just the two of you.

Focus group score: 87   Your score: ....

GREAT SEX POSITION NO. 5: THE RIDER

This is the first of the rear-entry positions. The woman lies face down on the bed with her legs together, but in order for the man to be able to penetrate she'll first have to raise her buttocks a little. Once he's in, she sinks down and, kneeling, he straddles her and sits down on her buttocks and upper thighs. He needs a strong erection, otherwise he's liable to get squeezed out. He's now sitting somewhat like a horse rider and, if you fit together well enough, by making the same kind of movements as if in a canter his glans will be jiggling the entrance of the vagina and G-spot, giving you both the most exquisite sensations. If you've never ridden a horse before don't worry – you'll soon work it out. Additional sensations can be created by you both using your PC muscles. She can rub her clitoris against the bed or, better still, against a vibrator, placed underneath and against her vulva. She can also bend one of her legs at the knee and use her heel to massage her partner's buttocks and anus – a cunning move which, if the man isn't expecting it, will provide an extremely pleasant surprise.

Focus group score: 86   Your score: ....

Variation 1. A couple of pillows can be placed under the woman's hips. This raises her vulva enough for the man to be able to thrust.

Focus group score: 82   Your score: ....

Variation 2. The woman reaches behind her to take hold of her own ankles. She then pulls her calves up and, by opposing the muscles of her arms and legs, curves her back into the shape of a bow. Because her hips are tilted her partner can enter her quite easily and the tension the position creates can quickly lead to orgasm.

Focus group score: 48   Your score: ....

GREAT SEX POSITION NO. 6:
THE SITTING EMBRACE

This, together with its variations, is the ultimate sex position for egalitarian couples. You face one another on more or less the same level, so there's no question of dominance and submission. It's comfortable and you can both move (the woman very easily) or you can stop moving for a time. You can chat. You can talk dirty. You can share fantasies. You can drink. You can eat. You can co-ordinate breathing (perhaps while blowing in one another's ears). And the man can give his partner just about every kind of stimulation that exists.

The man sits in the middle of the bed, either with his legs out straight or crossed. The woman now straddles him and lowers herself onto his penis. Squatting on her feet she can keep the penis and vagina in perfect alignment for a truly thrilling sensation. If she spreads her thighs widely she can increase the muscular tension as well as open her genitals to her lover's gaze and fingers. Better still, the man can take her buttocks in his hands, supporting her and guiding her movements, while his fingertips play with her labia and anus.

Focus group score: 85   Your score: ....

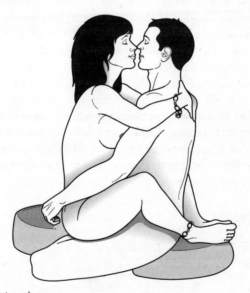

Figure 6.2 The Sitting embrace.

Variation 1. The woman kneels rather than squats, which is considerably less tiring but slightly less exciting.

Focus group score: 84   Your score: ....

Variation 2. No woman can keep either the main or the variation I position up for very long, no matter how much her man would like her to. For a rest she unfolds her legs so that, still sitting on his penis, she can put her feet around his back.

Focus group score: 79   Your score: ....

Variation 3. After experiencing the intimacy of variation for a while, the woman can lean away, throwing back her head, while her lover's hands behind her shoulders prevent her falling.

Focus group score: 68   Your score: ....

Variation 4. Now if the man leans back as well, and each of you holds the other's ankles or feet for support, you'll both be able to enjoy the view.

Focus group score: 61   Your score: ....

Variation 5. From variation 2 (the man with his ankles crossed and the woman with her legs behind his back) you take hold of one another's arms for support and both gradually lower yourselves until your heads are resting on the bed. Then pull yourselves up and repeat again and again, slowly, so that the resulting movement

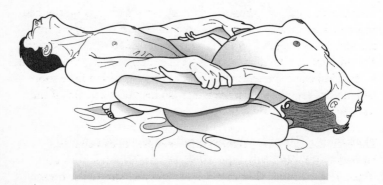

Figure 6.3 Mula Bandha.

creates friction between penis and vagina. In tantric sex this is known as *Mula Bandha*. If you want, you can remain in the lying down phase for long periods, your genitals locked together.

GREAT SEX POSITION NO. 7: CUDDLY BEARS

This is another rear-entry position. It's popularly known as 'the doggy' but since some people object to this, on the grounds that they don't want to have sex like dogs, I've renamed it Cuddly bears.

Of course, from the woman's point of view, a rear-entry position like this does allow a man to see *everything*. If you're shy about that and have never done it before, then try it first of all in the dark. There's also the likelihood of the vagina being pumped full of air – which, then, noisily escapes. On the plus side, this position allows for very deep penetration, excellent stimulation of the G-spot and a feeling of openness that can be very erotic. For the man, rear entry can be powerfully stimulating visually as well as providing plenty of ways for him to excite his partner, as you'll see in a moment.

Although it's fairly easy to achieve simultaneous orgasm by rear entry, it's probably more romantic to reserve that for a face-to-face position.

The essence of Cuddly bears is that the woman kneels on the bed and then rests her face sideways on a pillow, thus swinging the entrance to her vagina around so the man can enter from behind. The amount she opens her legs alters the height of her vulva as well as the sensations she feels. The man kneels or, with a little more athleticism, crouches with open legs (so his knees are out of the way) to increase his own tension.

The man can hold his partner's feet or hips. He can slap her buttocks (not too hard), separate them, tantalize her anus and slide a finger inside. He can reach around and stroke her breasts and nipples or, reaching further down, her clitoris. He can lean forwards and nuzzle her ears and she can even turn her face to kiss. He can take hold of her hair and bite her neck, which is, indeed, what other animals do. And very exciting it can be, but be gentle.

For a completely different set of sensations the man can lean well back and you can then both concentrate on your own genital feelings.

Focus group score: 84   Your score: ....

Variation 1. Instead of resting her face on a pillow, the woman can support herself on straight arms so that her back is more or less horizontal.

Focus group score: 81   Your score: ....

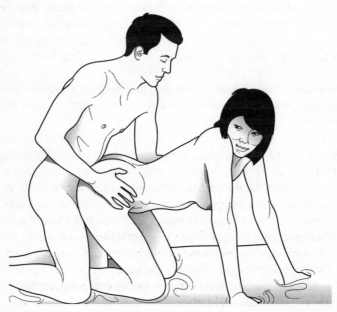

Figure 6.4 Cuddly bears.

Variation 2. Instead of kneeling, the man sits with his legs bent and open. The woman, on hands and knees, then reverses up to him until she can sink down.

Focus group score: 73   Your score: ....

Variation 3. The woman stands and puts her hands on a low support (the edge of the bed, the seat of a chair or a low table, for example). This is a lot more comfortable than variation 5.

Focus group score: 68   Your score: ....

Variation 4. The woman kneels half upright, supporting herself with her arms, but with her buttocks well clear of the bed. The man adopts a position as if sitting in the bucket seat of a sports car, with his legs out in front of him and holding himself up by his arms. He then 'drives' up to his partner, with one leg either side of her, until he can engage.

Focus group score: 58   Your score: ....

Variation 5. The woman stands and puts her hands on the floor. This is pretty tiring for most women.

Focus group score: 39   Your score: ....

Insight

You should already have located the G-spot and had a go at stimulating it with your fingers. If not, look again at Chapters 2 and 5. But how do you get at it with a penis? Since it's located on the front wall of the vagina, just inside the entrance, penetration is best from behind and not very deep. Only the glans of the penis should penetrate inside. Take hold of the base of your penis to exert extra pressure, or let your partner take hold of it.

GREAT SEX POSITION NO. 8: THE MISSIONARY REST POSITION

After you've enjoyed yourselves for a while in one of the missionary positions, there comes a point when you might want to take a breather, but without letting the excitement die down too much. Without disengaging, the man rolls onto his side, taking his partner with him. This is a nicely relaxed posture in which you can just do nothing for a while. When it's necessary to raise the temperature a little the man can make the occasional thrust. When it's necessary to raise the temperature a lot, he can lift his partner's upper leg for a view of her genitals and thrust more vigorously.

Focus group score: 79   Your score: ....

GREAT SEX POSITION NO. 9: TWO TRIANGLES

This is a position that makes you feel very athletic because of the way it opens and stretches the body, and yet it's very easy to do. It's also one of the positions in which you both feel equal. The man kneels and either sits on his feet or sits between his feet, whichever is most comfortable. He spreads his thighs and leans back a little, placing his hands on the ground behind him to help take the weight of his upper body. The woman now squats down onto her partner's penis and while sitting on his thighs also leans back, just as he is doing, taking her weight on her arms. It's a position with a lot of subtle variations. You can both vary how much you open or close your thighs, to help control the sexual tension, and also vary how much you lean back so that you can be close and intimate or, at the other extreme, feel more concentrated on your own personal feelings.

Focus group score: 76   Your score: ....

GREAT SEX POSITION NO. 10: THE CHAIR

This is, indeed, a position for a chair, and with the right design it can be immensely exciting. With the man sitting, the woman (facing him) steps up onto the chair, with her feet on the seat either side of her partner's buttocks. She then lowers herself onto him. If it's a chair without arms she can also straddle him with her feet on the floor. Swapping between these two positions, she can give her partner and herself very different sensations.

Focus group score: 75   Your score: ....

Variation 1. The woman faces away from the man.

Focus group score: 69   Your score: ....

GREAT SEX POSITION NO. 11: THE TRAP DOOR

The woman lies on her side. The man raises her upper leg and, facing her, kneels down to straddle her lower thigh. The view is exciting, he can feel her lower thigh against his buttocks,

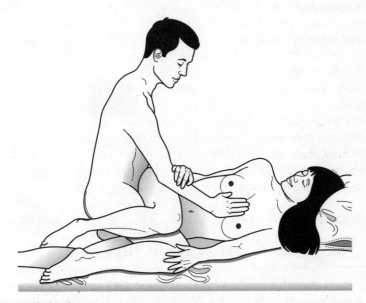

Figure 6.5 The Trap door.

penetration can be deep or shallow and he can either stroke her clitoris or let her do it.

Focus group score: 73   Your score: ....

GREAT SEX POSITION NO. 12: THE AMAZON

This position is similar to the Trap door except the roles are reversed and it's the woman who's in control. The man lies on his side. The woman raises his upper leg and, facing him, kneels down to straddle his lower thigh. Sliding forwards she engages. Here, she can control the depth of penetration and also rub her clitoris against his upper thigh.

Focus group score: 71   Your score: ....

GREAT SEX POSITION NO. 13: SPOONS

From the Rider position, just roll together onto your sides, without disengaging.

Focus group score: 70   Your score: ....

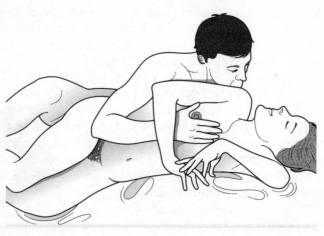

Figure 6.6 Spoons.

GREAT SEX POSITION NO. 14: AUTUMN DOG

One afternoon while having fun with my lover, I invented this position. Then I discovered it was the 26th position of the T'ung Hsüan Tzu (a famous Taoist text dating from the seventh century) known as Autumn dog. You *both* get on hands and knees and reverse up to one another. The man then swings his penis right around between his legs as far as it will go and inserts it. It needs a penis of at least average size and it works best with a taller man and a shorter woman, otherwise it's hard to get things aligned. Adopting the position for rear-entry sex is something that most women are used to but for men it can be novel. A man experiences the same sort of 'open' sensation that women get. For the woman, there's intense pressure on the G-spot from the penis because it's under tension. You can both reach between your legs to stimulate one another and yourselves or you can reach around behind and feel one another that way. **A word of warning:** It's better for the man not to ejaculate in this position as the penis is somewhat constricted.

Focus group score: 68   Your score: ....

Insight

Once again I'm going to emphasize the importance of lubrication, especially for older couples. For prolonged sessions, something additional is always necessary.
For advice on lubricants see Chapter 9.

GREAT SEX POSITION NO. 15: KALI ASANA

This position gets its name from the goddess, important in Tantra, who rides on a passive male. It's a position that quite decisively puts the woman in the dominant position because the man is lying on his back unable to do very much. 'Kali' then straddles him, on her knees, and pleasures herself.

Focus group score: 67   Your score: ....

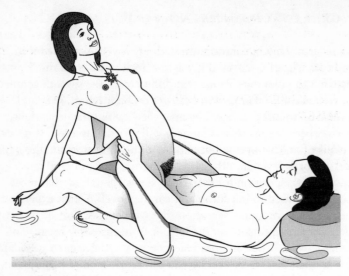

Figure 6.7 Kali asana.

Variation 1. If you have one of those benches without a back, or anything resembling it, the man can lie along it on his back and the woman can straddle both him and the bench. This is a great arrangement for a woman to go wild.

Focus group score: 67   Your score: ....

GREAT SEX POSITION NO. 16: THE SWING

If you have children you've probably got a swing in the garden. If not, you may have a swinging seat in the house. If not, get one. There are various ways of going about things. The easiest is for the woman to sit on the seat and for the man to stand or kneel, depending on height. It can be very languid. The woman can also lie over the seat.

Focus group score: 66   Your score: ....

Variation 1. Get two swings.

Focus group score: n/a (nobody had two swings)

Your score: ....

GREAT SEX POSITION NO. 17: THE REVERSE MISSIONARY

Just like the Missionary, but in this case it's the woman who's lying on top.

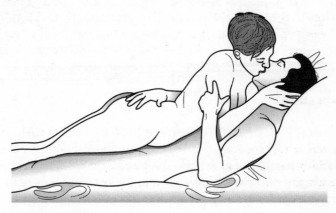

Figure 6.8 The Reverse missionary.

Focus group score: 66

Your score: ....

GREAT SEX POSITION NO. 18: HIGH HEELS

This is the first of the standing positions. It's face to face and an exciting precursor to the main action if you get carried away in, say, the kitchen or somewhere out of doors.

It's called High heels because, depending on relative heights, the woman usually needs to be taller and high heels (especially worn with nothing else) are an excellent solution. Or one of you may have to stand on a step. Even with the woman's legs well apart it can be difficult for her partner to penetrate and it helps a lot if the woman wraps a leg around the man. It also helps to have something to lean against.

Focus group score: 65   Your score: ....

GREAT SEX POSITION NO. 19: THE SCISSORS

It's probably easiest to get into this position by toppling sideways from the Rider. The woman, now lying on her side, straightens her legs so they pass either side of her partner's waist, like a pair of scissors to cut him in half. Meanwhile, the man, also on his side, still engaged and between her legs, now straightens his legs and bends at the waist to bring his feet towards his lover's face. It's an unusual angle of entry that can produce interesting sensations.

Focus group score: 64   Your score: ....

GREAT SEX POSITION NO. 20: THE MAGIC CARPET

With the man lying on his back, the woman sits on him, facing, cross-legged or if she can manage it, in the yoga lotus position.

Focus group score: 63   Your score: ....

Variation 1. Instead of sitting cross-legged, the woman sits with her legs out straight, her feet either side of her partner's head.

Focus group score: 57   Your score: ....

Variation 2. Instead of facing her partner, the woman faces sideways.

Focus group score: 55   Your score: ....

Variation 3. The woman faces her partner's feet.

Focus group score: 54   Your score: ....

GREAT SEX POSITION NO. 21: PASSERS BY

The easiest way of getting into this position is from the Magic
carpet, variation 1. The woman puts both feet one side of her
partner's head. She then topples sideways, without disengaging,
taking her lover with her. The man is now lying on his side, with
his partner's heels close to his face. The woman remains well bent
at the waist. Both of you can rest on your elbows and be relaxed.
It's a position of detachment, good for cooling down a little, but the
woman can always stimulate her own clitoris for greater excitement.

Focus group score: 62   Your score: ....

GREAT SEX POSITION NO. 22: THE T

The woman lies on her back, then bends her knees and pulls them
back to her chest with her calves and feet in the air. The man lies
sideways across her thighs.

Focus group score: 60   Your score: ....

GREAT SEX POSITION NO. 23: THE DOUBLE-REVERSE MISSIONARY

With the man lying on his back, the woman lies on top but, unlike
the reverse missionary, she faces his feet. This is a curious position
that allows the woman to rub her clitoris against her partner's
scrotum.

Focus group score: 59   Your score: ....

GREAT SEX POSITION NO. 24: THE HAMMOCK

If you have a hammock, the woman can sit on the edge of it and
have sex just as for a swing, but, better still, the man can lie in it
face up while she straddles him with her feet on the ground

Focus group score: 59   Your score: ....

GREAT SEX POSITION NO. 25: WOMAN'S REVENGE

Men are always trying to get women into difficult positions. Here's one that turns the tables. Lying on his back, the man bends his legs and draws his knees up to his chest, his calves and feet sticking up in the air. In other words, he's in a similar position to the one the woman would be in for the Ball. The woman, facing him, now sits down on his buttocks and the backs of his thighs.

Focus group score: 57   Your score: ....

GREAT SEX POSITION NO. 26: CUDDLY KOALAS

The woman kneels beside the bed then leans across it – a variant on Cuddly bears. The man, also kneeling, enters from behind.

Focus group score: 56   Your score: ....

GREAT SEX POSITION NO. 27: ON THE EDGE

The woman lies on her back on the bed with her vulva at the edge. She can let her legs hang down or her partner, kneeling or standing depending on the height of the bed, can lift them up onto his shoulders.

Focus group score: 55   Your score: ....

GREAT SEX POSITION NO. 28: THE SUSPENSION BRIDGE

The woman lies face up with only her head and shoulders supported by the bed and her feet on the floor. The man kneels or stands between her thighs, depending on the height of the bed.

Focus group score: 53   Your score: ....

GREAT SEX POSITION NO. 29: THE STOOL

The woman sits on the stool and the man enters standing. She could also sit on a table, a kitchen work surface, a chair or anything handy.

Focus group score: 52   Your score: ....

Variation 1. The woman, face down, lies over the stool or kneels on the seat of the chair, leaning over the back for support. The man, kneeling or standing as appropriate, enters from behind.

Focus group score: 51   Your score: ....

GREAT SEX POSITION NO. 30: THE WALL

This is another standing position. Men like the idea of it, but it's pretty demanding for both partners. The woman puts her arms around her partner's neck and he lifts and supports her with his hands under her buttocks. It helps if the man leans against a wall, because the woman can then put her feet against it.

Focus group score: 50   Your score: ....

GREAT SEX POSITION NO. 31: THREE CHAIRS

The woman sits on one chair with her legs well apart, and one foot resting on each of the other two chairs, while the man kneels or stands. This is an excellent arrangement for a woman who can't take the weight of her partner on top.

Focus group score: 49   Your score: ....

GREAT SEX POSITION NO. 32: HIDE AND SEEK

This is an extraordinary position because the man has sex almost without seeing his partner at all, hence the name. The woman lies on her back with her hips raised almost vertically by a pile of cushions, so that she's in roughly the same position as for the Exhibitionist (No. 3). A couch can be better than a bed because the woman's hips can then be supported by the armrest. The man engages facing *away* from her. He can focus entirely on his sensations, which can be intensified by his partner giving him a few slaps on the buttocks.

Focus group score: 48   Your score: ....

GREAT SEX POSITION NO. 33: THE GYMNAST

If you have anything in your home from which you can hang (an exercise bar, a door frame, or a tree in the garden), the woman can swing on it, wrapping her legs around the man for support.

Focus group score: 46   Your score: ....

GREAT SEX POSITION NO. 34: THE WHEELBARROW

Standing facing the bed, the woman leans onto it with straight arms and places her knees on the edge of the mattress. The man, standing behind, takes hold of her legs just below the knees and lifts her. The woman needs strong arms, otherwise she's liable to collapse.

Focus group score: 40   Your score: ....

GREAT SEX POSITION NO. 35: DRILLING FOR OIL

Some positions, like this one, just can't be taken very seriously, but they're good fun. If you can learn to be sufficiently uninhibited to at least give them a try, then the whole of your 'serious' lovemaking will be enhanced by that freedom.

The woman does a shoulder stand. That is, from a lying down position she first raises her legs and then her hips until her back is vertical. She can hold herself in position with her hands on her sides and lower back. She then opens her legs so the man stands astride between them.

Variation 1. The woman folds her legs down, but keeping her feet clear of her vulva, in which case the man can straddle her in either direction.

Focus group score: 36   Your score: ....

Switching positions

A word about switching postures. There's absolutely no reason at all that you shouldn't break apart for a major change in position. As we've seen, this is the traditional Arab technique of *imsak*, for prolonging sex. But it can also be fun to try to move as seamlessly as possible from one position to the next without disengaging. For example, you can roll from a man-on-top posture to a woman-on-top, and then back again...and back again. A thickly carpeted floor is excellent because it gives you the space to roll over and over. Otherwise, have the biggest bed you can afford and have room for. See if you can work out how to get from a rear-entry position into a face-to-face position without disengaging. The key to it all is a powerful erection (otherwise the penis is liable to slip out when you move) and a talent for three-dimensional visualization.

Sex out of doors

Sex out of doors can be very special. You can be doing something exciting that makes your body feel so alive that you just *have* to have sex. Maybe it happens when you're jogging together, or riding, or skiing, or swimming to an isolated cove or deserted island.

The problem is *how* to do it when you don't have a bed, a chair or even a cushion, and the ground is hard, uneven, stony or scratchy.

Standing up is one solution. Another is for the woman to bend over and take hold of, say, a convenient rock or tree, while the man enters from behind. The sitting embrace can work quite well because only the man's buttocks need to be in hard contact with the ground and they can be protected by throwing some clothes down. Or maybe you can find a convenient rock or tree stump to sit on. Other possibilities include Two triangles, Autumn dog and variations 2 and 3 of Cuddly bears.

For positions to use during pregnancy see Chapter 12.

Positions for anal sex

Since the anus is very close to the entrance to the vagina, then, logically, anal intercourse should be possible in just about any of the positions used for vaginal intercourse. But the anus is generally a lot harder to get into than the vagina and some positions make it more difficult still by creating tension and obscuring the target. Probably the best position for anal beginners is Cuddly bears (No. 7) because it gives a man a clear view of where he's headed. The snag with it is that it can cause the anus to contract. To overcome that, the woman can lie flat as in the Rider (No. 5) but with her legs somewhat apart; to help, she can easily reach behind and spread her buttocks. The Improved missionary (No. 1) results in a more relaxed anus, while the Ball (No. 2) and the Exhibitionist (No. 3) make it easy for a man to see what he's doing. Of course, there's no reason a woman can't also take control of things. The Sitting embrace (No. 6) and the Chair (No. 10) allow her to lower herself onto her man and thus control the depth of penetration – but that requires quite a lot of skill since nobody can see what's going on.

10 THINGS TO REMEMBER

1 *There are at least 10 good reasons to try lots of different positions, including varying the muscular tension, the area and intensity of stimulation, and the emotional effect.*

2 *Positions that create muscular tension are most likely to lead to whole body orgasms.*

3 *In my focus groups, the well-known missionary position, improved with the help of a nice, thick pillow, remains the most popular position.*

4 *In total there are 35 positions in this chapter for you to try, together with 32 variations.*

5 *Face-to-face positions create the greatest intimacy.*

6 *Rear-entry positions are more detached but give good stimulation to the G-spot; you can also take hold of the penis and press it against the G-spot.*

7 *Unless you're happy always playing the same roles, you should each have the opportunity to be dominant and in control; for equality try the sitting embrace.*

8 *There's no reason you shouldn't disengage between positions but it can also be fun to string several positions together while keeping the penis firmly in the vagina.*

9 *Even in the most unpromising outdoor terrain, sex is always possible if you're inventive (try the Sitting embrace or the Wall).*

10 *The easiest positions for anal intercourse are those that relax the muscles and also allow a clear view.*

HOW GREAT IS SEX NOW?

▸ *Have you tried at least six new positions?*　　　　Yes/No

▸ *Have you included man-dominant, woman-dominant and equal positions?*　　　　Yes/No

▸ *Have you tried at least two rear-entry positions?*　　　　Yes/No

▸ *Have you been completely uninhibited?*　　　　Yes/No

▸ *Have you tried sharing food and drink during intercourse?*　　　　Yes/No

▸ *Have you used furniture other than the bed?*　　　　Yes/No

▸ *Have you been topping up the lubricant from time to time?*　　　　Yes/No

▸ *Have you managed to run through a sequence of positions without disengaging?*　　　　Yes/No

▸ *Have you had sex out of doors?*　　　　Yes/No

▸ *Have you tried anal intercourse in at least two positions?*　　　　Yes/No

If you answered 'no' to more than three questions, re-read the relevant parts of the chapter and make an effort to put the suggestions into effect. There's nothing wrong with the Missionary position and, if you're like most people, you'll use it a lot. But it can be improved. What's more, a variety of positions not only keeps sex interesting and stimulating but allows you to take turns at being in control.

7

....

Great sex is in the mind

In this chapter you will learn:
- *how to communicate excitement*
- *that words are the most powerful aphrodisiac*
- *how fantasies can intensify arousal and orgasm*
- *how sex can be spiritual as well as physical.*

So far I've said very little about the body's most important sex organ. It lies not between the thighs but between the ears. It is, of course, the brain, and it is the subject of this chapter.

Orgasm really occurs in the brain. Of course, there are all the physical signs of orgasm that we've already talked about, but what really count are the electrical changes in the brain and the neurochemical changes that take place in the part known as the 'limbic system'. If you don't believe it, reflect on the fact that men who have had their spinal cords severed in accidents can still have erections and can still ejaculate (and father children), *but they feel nothing*. The feeling of orgasm requires the brain.

The limbic system is one of the most primitive parts of the 1,360 g (3 lb) of cells and juices that make you, you. Millions of years ago, our ancestors already had it. In other words, the limbic system is *animal*. If you want to excite your partner, you mainly have to deal in 'animal' things. This is probably why women in the twenty-first century can still be aroused by a bite on the neck.

What goes on in the brain?

What is actually going on in the brain when we feel sexually aroused? For one thing, the electrical activity in our brains changes. When we're awake, we are usually in what is known as the 'Beta state'. That is to say, the dominant frequency of our brains is at its highest: we're alert and ready for any action that might be necessary. For sex (and meditation), we want to get into the 'Alpha state', which is at a slightly lower frequency. We're still fully awake but also very relaxed.

Table 3 Brain waves.

State	Frequency	Description
Delta	0.5–4.0 Hz	Deep sleep
Theta	4.0–8.0 Hz	Drowsiness/light sleep
Alpha	**8.0–14 Hz**	**Awake but relaxed**
Beta	14–30 Hz	Awake and alert

Many other changes take place in the brain during sex. The amplitude of something called the 'p300 brain waves' drops sharply. These are the brain's normal responses to anything at all, arriving 300 milliseconds after an event. Activity falls in the amygdala and hippocampus, areas concerned with alertness and anxiety and, when orgasm comes, activity falls in the prefrontal cortex, too. In other words, certain brain activity shuts down.

At the same time, there are changes in neurochemical activity, which we already looked at in Chapter 2. The result of all this is that there will come a point when you feel that your brain alters its state of consciousness as clearly as if someone had moved a switch. One moment your perception of things around you is normal; you don't really feel 'turned on' even though you may be starting to have sex. Then, suddenly, 'ping', the switch is thrown, and you're no longer aware of anything but the two of you. You have the feeling of climbing inside your own brain and saying goodbye to the world.

One of the neurochemicals is dopamine. Essentially, you get a 'fix' of a substance naturally produced by the body that induces ecstasy.

....

Insight

You can prolong your dopamine 'hit' by sharing a glass of wine with your partner *after* sex. Don't drink much alcohol before sex because it reduces performance. But a *little* alcohol after sex has the effect of inhibiting the breakdown of dopamine and therefore of extending the glow that follows lovemaking.

....

When you only use physical techniques in lovemaking, you bring all these changes about *indirectly*. However, there are ways of working *directly* inside the brain itself. That's what we're going to learn about next.

GET RID OF NEGATIVE EMOTIONS

The limbic system is extremely powerful. It can completely take over and make you do things that your more logical neocortex would never do. Nevertheless, it also has its weaknesses. One of them is that the sexual response in the brain is prey to all kinds of anxieties and negative emotions that can intrude and spoil things. If you have any 'issues' with your partner, use our old friend *communication* to deal with them before the next sex session.

Anxieties about the relationship, about work, about the children and so on are all passion killers, and the impact appears to be even greater on women than on men. Yet there's another category of anxiety that can be very negative, and it seems to affect men more than women; anxiety about sexual performance.

As many men know, fear that the penis may not work properly almost guarantees that it won't. If the problem is in the mind, then the answer is to use the mind to cure itself. This works equally well for whatever anxieties a woman may have too. Visualize, whenever you can, having sex successfully. This is a little bit of self-hypnosis. Let's say that you are anxious about your erection:

- ▶ *Visualize blood flowing into your penis and your penis becoming erect.*
- ▶ *Visualize how hard and handsome it is.*
- ▶ *Visualize your partner's excitement at seeing it.*
- ▶ *Visualize entering your partner.*
- ▶ *Visualize her pleasure at the feel of you.*

The technique won't work in a single session; these kinds of visualizations need to be repeated over and over. Similarly, you can use visualization to work out a new position or technique so that you'll feel more confident when you try it.

THE ZONE

When athletes particularly excel, they call the experience 'flow' or the 'zone'. This is when they achieve more than they ever have before and they cannot explain it. It can happen again and again, but it's very difficult to bring it about deliberately, which is why sports psychologists can earn a lot of money. In sex, too, you can be in the 'zone'. That, in fact, is what you're aiming for. It's a state in which all of your attention is focused on a very narrow band of experience. You're not aware of the outside world, you're not aware of the room, you're not aware of the bed, and you're probably not even aware of all of your partner. You're only aware of what your partner is doing and what you're doing, and you feel a sense of ecstasy as you do it.

I've said that you cannot deliberately enter the zone, but you can do a few things to make it more likely:

- ▶ *Concentrate intensely on what you're doing and don't think of anything else.*
- ▶ *Make sure there can be no distractions. Disconnect the telephone, for example.*

▶ *Do something just slightly 'harder' than you ever have before. Things that are too routine don't evoke flow. On the other hand, things that provoke performance anxiety also work against flow.*

While you're trying out the ideas in this book, you probably won't find it easy to get into the zone. You'll quite likely be too distracted by checking the instructions. Don't worry about it. Once you've incorporated the things that appeal to you into your lovemaking, you'll quickly get into the right frame of mind.

Have a go
Are there any 'artificial' things that you can do to help you enter the zone? Yes, there are. Try making love to music and try without music. Music (assuming you like it) stimulates the reward structures in your brain, such as the part known as the 'ventral tegmental area'. This is exactly the same area that sex itself activates. In other words, with the right music you already have a head start. At the same time, activity in the amygdala, the part of the brain associated with fear, is reduced. You could also watch a sexy film (see Chapter 9). Another and very powerful way, as you'll see later in the chapter, is to use fantasy.

Insight
During intercourse, take hold of your partner's head with your palms resting lightly and your fingertips spread out. Make sure you don't cover the ears. Now, think how much you love your partner and send that message directly to his or her brain through your fingertips as they wiggle gently over the scalp.

Body language

The first form of communication is body language. It is, of course, the principal language of many animals, and quite effective, too. In fact, some experts say that about three-quarters of all the messages we send are in the form of body language, which means that other animals can communicate about three-quarters as well as human beings.

In society, we're quite restrained in our use of body language, and we're not very good at interpreting it either. Nonetheless, we all know and understand expressions like 'you could cut the atmosphere with a knife'. Nobody is saying anything but, from body language, we subconsciously know that something is wrong.

You can certainly tell if you partner is excited or not, even if nothing at all is said. You can see and feel. Even in the dark, there's a kind of electricity in the air when things are going well and a kind of flat feeling when they're not.

So, whether you're a man or a woman, don't just – man or woman – lie there 'and think of England'. What kinds of things can you do?

▶ *Tear at your own clothes.*
▶ *Tear at your partner's clothes.*
▶ *Allow your mouth to open.*
▶ *Suck your fingers.*
▶ *Pull faces.*
▶ *Run your hands all over your body.*
▶ *Massage your own breasts and nipples.*
▶ *Move your hips.*
▶ *Open your legs.*

In other words, just let yourself go. Let's just remember why: apart from the fact that you're getting 'lost' in sex, which is good, you're trying to make your partner excited simply by being excited yourself.

No more silent sex

In my focus groups, I was surprised to discover how many couples *don't* talk when they're having sex. If that sounds like you, it's perhaps because you feel words will somehow destroy the 'magic'.

Yet sex can be much more exciting when you moan and groan, and especially when you *do* talk.

Nothing can excite a partner so much as the way you express your own excitement. 'Talking dirty' is an art that all lovers should master. Of course, that doesn't mean, as in the old joke, telling your partner that the ceiling needs painting. Nor do you have to have the poetic talents of Shakespeare. So what exactly *do* you say?

First of all, you want your partner to know when he or she is or isn't doing the right thing. 'That's exactly the right place.' 'A bit lower.' 'Faster.' Compliment your partner when it's good, rather than criticize when it's bad. 'The pressure you used just then was perfect.'

Second, you need to be sure *you're* doing the right thing. 'Here?' 'Faster?' 'Slower?' Admittedly, these kinds of questions would get a little tedious if you had to ask them every time. But you won't; next time you'll know.

So, that's communicating information. Now let's take a look at communicating excitement. Sounds are part of this: moans, groans, sighs, screams, yells, pants, sobs.

Words are even more powerful and, for most people, this works all the better if you use the 'dirtiest' words. They're far more exciting than the dictionary words. Just say whatever comes into your head. Put words to your feelings. Obviously, try not to use words you know your partner objects to. On the other hand, during the excitement, different standards can apply. If nothing *does* immediately come into your head here are some suggestions:

▶ *Describe how excited your partner is making you.*
▶ *Describe what you're going to do to your partner.*
▶ *Tell your partner how you want him or her to lie or sit or kneel, etc.*
▶ *Say what it is about your partner that turns you on.*
▶ *Tell your partner what you want him or her to do to you.*
▶ *Describe the stage of excitement you've reached.*

Fantasy – the ultimate aphrodisiac

Some people say that they don't fantasize at all. Well, if you don't then you *should*! Fantasies, and especially fantasies spoken aloud, whether during masturbation or sex with a partner, are probably the most powerful aphrodisiacs that exist. (In fact, they can be too powerful, bringing lovemaking to an all too quick climax.)

FANTASIES WHILE MASTURBATING

If you haven't yet discovered fantasizing for yourself, masturbate in your normal way without fantasy. After a while, continue masturbating while visualizing the sexiest scene you can imagine. Almost immediately you'll notice an increase in your excitement.

Fantasizing while masturbating is wonderful. You don't have to worry about upsetting a partner. You don't have to worry about being thought weird. There's just you and your imagination. You can be with any film star you choose, any friend or acquaintance, any number of people, in any place, doing anything you like.

Use props if you like. Men often like to use their partners' underwear to help them visualize that they're actually there.

Now say something aloud, as if, for example, addressing someone in your fantasy. Be as 'dirty' as you wish. Perhaps say something you've never dared say before. You may orgasm straight away, or be very close to doing so.

FANTASY AS THERAPY

As I mentioned in Chapter 1, visualization can be a great form of therapy. By imagining things you're anxious about you can overcome repression.

Suppose, for example, that your partner wants to perform oral sex on you and that, while secretly you think you might like it, you just can't bring yourself to permit it. As soon as your partner moves down there, you freeze. This is the sort of situation where fantasy may help. In the comfort and security of your bedroom, on your own, you can run through a scenario involving oral sex. Break the whole thing down into a series of steps. Like this:

▶ *My partner arouses my genitals with fingers.*
▶ *My partner lubricates my genitals with fingers moistened with saliva.*
▶ *My partner dribbles saliva directly onto my genitals.*
▶ *My partner brushes my genitals with his or her lips.*
▶ *My partner brushes my genitals with his or her tongue.*
▶ *My partner takes my genitals into his or her mouth.*
▶ *My partner makes me orgasm.*

Begin masturbating while visualizing the first step. If you're comfortable with that, move to the next stage. If you reach a stage with which you feel anxious, return to the previous one and masturbate to orgasm while fantasizing about that. During the orgasm, move forward to the stage that made you anxious. Essentially it's a process of desensitizing and, at the same time, reward (the pleasure of orgasm). Over a period of days or weeks, continue the therapy until you feel happy and relaxed about the whole thing.

FANTASY WITH A PARTNER

You might consider that sexual fantasies are unhealthy, a sign of problems within a relationship or a retreat into a make-believe world rather than the creation of an exciting real world. Well, that *could* be the case, but it all depends on the fantasies. There's a huge difference between, say, fantasizing that you and your partner are the star attractions at a sex show, and really wishing your partner was somebody else when making love. Fantasies can be extremely positive. Once you start sharing fantasies, you're laying bare your partner's mind and soul. You're going deeper and getting more intimate than ever before. Fantasies can:

▶ *raise the level of excitement*
▶ *short-cut arousal*
▶ *go straight to the relevant parts of the brain*
▶ *reveal things about your partner that you never knew before*
▶ *increase the sense of intimacy between you*
▶ *introduce ideas you can go on to use in reality if you wish.*

A private fantasy, as opposed to a joint fantasy, is certainly not a recipe for better sex with a partner. A fantasy that you're not willing to share is best reserved for daydreams and masturbation. It will simply distract you from your partner. A fantasy shared, on the other hand, is a recipe for great sex.

At one end of the spectrum, you might simply introduce a fantasy about something that you'd like to do together but have never dared mention before. During the excitement of sex, for example, you might 'confess' that you once had a dream about licking and sucking your partner's genitals and that in this dream your partner was driven wild. At the other end of the spectrum might come a totally impossible fantasy involving, say, a harem of 100 women.

Sexual fantasies are no different to the TV programmes where everyone lives in luxurious mansions, drives fast cars and has shiny, white teeth. Everything is equally perfect. Nobody refuses anything. Nobody has any sexual problems. Nobody is jealous or resentful or hurt. Nobody has omitted to wash or has bad breath or any sexually transmitted diseases. There are no consequences and no messy entanglements afterwards. Clearly, most fantasies could never become reality simply because they are, by definition, just that – unreal. Nevertheless, fantasies may open the door to real-life experimentation – if you *want* them to. Equally, there's no reason why they can't remain in the world of the intangible if you prefer.

Try to find out what your partner's sexual fantasies are. At first, this might be delicate. Fantasies can blow your mind but they can also blow up your relationship if you start on a subject your partner is frightened about. Proceed gently. You could begin by introducing a fantasy that you believe your partner will find exciting. Just hint at a subject during sex and see if he or she responds. Here are some ideas:

▶ *I wish I could have been in your changing room today with all those women/men.*
▶ *Last night I dreamed we were making love on a beach and people were watching.*
▶ *Last night I dreamed we were at an orgy.*

If your partner doesn't take up the idea, don't press it. Try again another day after the concept has had time to sink in. If he or she responds, then you can take turns to progress the story, prompting one another and carrying on the narrative. You may find out unexpected things about yourself and your partner too.

It sometimes happens that the one to introduce fantasy into lovemaking is then shocked by a partner's response. Suddenly, you could be confronted by ideas you weren't expecting and that you find difficult to deal with. You may feel that by unlocking these fantasies you've encouraged behaviour that, in the real world, would be devastating to you. Relax. This is unlikely to be the case. Remember that your partner has always had these fantasies. The only difference is that now you know about them too.

Insight
Your partner will feel relieved and probably even exhilarated when his or her fantasies are in the open. Better sex is all about the freedom to be yourself in the presence of another person. By expressing your innermost thoughts and feelings, and allowing your partner to do the same, you're taking sex to its highest level.

What kinds of things are we talking about? Well, women often fantasize about being watched. There is, after all, an exhibitionist streak in many women so it's hardly surprising if that's also an element in their fantasies. Women may like to imagine someone watching while they're undressing or sunbathing in the nude or masturbating or making love. Another aspect of women's fantasies is being forced to do something (in the nicest possible way). This has to do with the notion of being absolved of guilt. In other words, the fantasy might involve being tied up by a film star and then ordered to perform fellatio. Incidentally, if your partner wants you to pretend to be James Bond or George Clooney, take it as a compliment.

Men often fantasize about being in bed with their partners and another woman. Maybe one of their partner's friends, for example. Or they fantasize about a woman acquaintance, or about sexual techniques they've never tried – anal sex, for example. More than women, men are likely to fantasize about tying up and spanking and that sort of thing.

If these kinds of subjects just don't seem to go with your style of sex, then find fantasies that do. You can equally fantasize about sex on a deserted beach, on a mountain top or even in the clouds.

Insight

When you've found a fantasy that really turns your partner on, it's tempting to keep repeating it. But, if you do, it'll gradually lose its power. So, while sticking with the same successful theme come up with new ideas each time – a different place, different people, different circumstances and so on.

Introducing fantasy is like a direct line into the brain. It can cause arousal far faster than any physical technique. Once you're 'up there', you don't necessarily have to continue the fantasy any further. Nor should you use fantasy every time. Treat it like other techniques. Not something to be used repetitively, but part of the range of things you can do.

Spiritual sex

So far in this chapter, I've concentrated on ways in which the brain and the mind can enhance physical sensation. But there is another side to this – the way the chemicals generated by the physical body and brain during sex can lead to intensely spiritual experiences in the mind. Tantra, which originated in India at least one and a half millennia ago, is probably the oldest tradition of using sex for spiritual purposes. Tantrikas believed that sex could be a way of arousing the divine energy stored within the body and of reaching a state of bliss that was a foretaste of the bliss that was to come as part of the great Oneness.

In my focus groups about half of the people say they have never felt anything spiritual during sex, while the other half say they've sometimes felt a spiritual connection with their partners; but only around one in ten reported ever feeling a spiritual connection with the whole universe. My focus groups are only a relatively small sample, of course, but those results suggest that a lot of people are missing out on optimum sex.

What does a spiritual experience feel like? Some people say that the physical and mental boundaries between themselves and their partners seem to soften and almost dissolve. They hardly know where their own body ends and their partner's body begins. The more rare spiritual experiences produce a profound sense of tranquility, a glow, a radiance; a sense that above the concerns of everyday life is a higher realm of bliss.

These kinds of phenomena are far more likely to occur during prolonged sex sessions when the build-up of chemicals results in a significantly altered state of consciousness. That means multiple orgasms for both women and men, which is the subject of the next chapter.

Insight

When you're having sex, try to co-ordinate your breathing. This is easiest in a position in which your heads are close together so that you can actually hear one another. To get into step, one of you may have to speed up a little and the other may have to slow down. Don't just do it for a few breaths; keep it up. Gradually, you'll have the sense of dissolving into one body and one mind.

10 THINGS TO REMEMBER

1 *The brain is the body's most important sex organ.*

2 *Significant changes take place in the brain during sex.*

3 *By using the power of the mind, we can influence the changes in the brain directly.*

4 *It's important to clear the mind of negative emotions before sex.*

5 *Intense concentration can take you into the 'zone'.*

6 *Use body language to communicate excitement to your partner.*

7 *Co-ordinate breathing to accentuate the feeling of oneness.*

8 *Talk 'dirty' during sex.*

9 *Fantasy is the ultimate aphrodisiac.*

10 *Great sex always has a spiritual dimension.*

HOW GREAT IS SEX NOW?

▶ *Have you entered an altered state of consciousness during sex?*   Yes/No

▶ *Have you rid yourself of negative emotions through communication and visualization?*   Yes/No

▶ *Have you got into the 'zone'?*   Yes/No

▶ *Have you been communicating passion through body language?*   Yes/No

▶ *Have you been telling your partner what you want during sex?*   Yes/No

▶ *Have you explored fantasy as a way of increasing excitement during masturbation?*   Yes/No

▶ *Have you explored fantasy as a way of dealing with inhibitions?*   Yes/No

▶ *Have you been sharing fantasies with your partner during sex?*   Yes/No

▶ *Have you had a spiritual experience during sex?*   Yes/No

If you answered 'no' to more than three questions, re-read the relevant parts of the chapter and make an effort to put the suggestions into effect. When it comes to sex, the brain can seem a rather boring sideshow. But, in reality, the physical body is really only a route to the mind. Playing the body is, in a way, like using the keyboard of a computer; what counts is what's happening in the processor. If you ignore the mind, you'll never take sex to its ultimate level.

8

....

Great multiple orgasms

In this chapter you will learn:
- *how women can have multiple orgasms*
- *how men can have multiple orgasms*
- *how to co-ordinate your orgasms.*

Until the mid-nineteenth century it was widely believed that women couldn't orgasm *at all*. Now, over 90 per cent of women experience orgasm, and the focus has moved instead to multiple orgasms. Men have become jealous. If women can have multiple orgasms, why can't men? Well, in fact, using a special technique, they can, as you'll see in this chapter.

Multiple orgasms for women

What, exactly, are 'multiple orgasms' in women? The famous sex researcher Shere Hite defines *multiple* orgasm in women as meaning closely repeated but distinct sets of muscular contractions. Orgasms separated by a few minutes are something different and Hite calls them 'sequential orgasms'. As far as I'm concerned (and according to the women in my focus groups), orgasms that come within seconds or minutes of one another are all multiples and are all great.

Some researchers say that about 15 per cent of women have multiple orgasms, some say 25 per cent and some say even higher.

Can you become one of them? At least one study suggests that heredity has at least something to do with it, so ask your mother if you dare. However, just as most women 'magically' became orgasmic during the second half of the twentieth century, so most women will become multi-orgasmic over the next few years. Of course, magic has nothing to do with it, it's much more a question of culture.

Years ago, women didn't have orgasms because they didn't *expect* to have orgasms (nor did their partners expect them to). Now, the majority of women have one orgasm because they expect to have just one orgasm. Some of them, it has to be said, are completely satisfied by their single orgasm and that's fine. But if you're not, then the first thing is to *believe* that you can be multi-orgasmic. In fact, you almost certainly are multi-orgasmic and you just don't know it. The way to unlock your multi-orgasmic capacity is not through intercourse but through masturbation. Sex with a partner can wait until you're reliably multi-orgasmic on your own.

In my focus groups, some women talk of having to 'work' at their orgasms. They sometimes describe their efforts as 'desperate' and 'grubby'. One woman said she had managed a second orgasm but it had taken 'too long'. When I asked how long, she said '15 minutes'. These women all have an attitude problem. If you think spending 15 minutes on sex is 'too long' then you're never going to enjoy yourself.

Take note, too, of the word 'grubby'. If you're going to become multi-orgasmic, you have to get rid of any negative attitudes like this and, instead, celebrate masturbation.

When masturbating you should be:

- *joyful*
- *uninhibited*
- *expansive*
- *inventive*
- *relaxed.*

Have a go

Have your one orgasm by your usual method of masturbation, but don't have it in the back of your mind that you'll settle for one if necessary. Be optimistic. Now simply continue to play with your clitoris. It may be that you'll surprise yourself by having a second orgasm without doing anything else. And a third.

If not, you're going to have to do something unusual, something extra, to get those additional orgasms. Later on, special techniques may not be necessary. In fact, women who are multi-orgasmic say that, after the first, orgasms come more easily. For now, while you're training your body to produce multiple orgasms, you may have to throw everything at it, up to but not quite including the kitchen sink. In Chapter 7 we looked at the power of the mind – use that to help you. Essentially you have to raise the erotic temperature higher than you ever have before and continue longer than you ever have before. Don't forget, either, that, as you saw in Chapter 2, orgasm is a release of tension. Before you can release that tension you first of all have to build it. Here are a few ideas:

- ▶ *Put on some sensual, very rhythmic music.*
- ▶ *Strip completely naked, if you're not already.*
- ▶ *Relax. Give yourself an hour to succeed.*
- ▶ *Rub yourself all over with some body oil while continuing to masturbate with your other hand.*
- ▶ *Use a vibrator (see Chapter 9).*
- ▶ *Try different positions. On your back, open your legs as far as you can or, alternatively, press them hard together with the vibrator between your thighs and against your vulva. Or try kneeling with your thighs open and lean back as far as you can – use some pillows to support you. The more physical tension you create the better.*
- ▶ *Use fantasy, as described in Chapter 7.*
- ▶ *Speak your fantasy out loud.*
- ▶ *Focus.*
- ▶ *Make plenty of noise.*

If you still haven't achieved further orgasms:

▶ *stimulate other places in addition to your clitoris – the entrance to your vagina, your G-spot area, your anus, your nipples – whatever excites you*
▶ *increase the blood flow by spanking yourself*
▶ *try masturbating while watching an erotic video or DVD*
▶ *try masturbating in front of a mirror or while making a video of yourself or watching yourself on a TV monitor (for how see Chapter 9).*

Don't stop until you've had at least three orgasms.

PROBLEMS

Some women report that they'd like to carry on stimulating themselves and believe they would have further orgasms but their clitorises becomes too sensitive to touch after the first orgasm. If this happens to you, try continuing the stimulation above your clitoris or to the side or try some of your other erogenous places. Above all, continue the stimulation in your mind. If you still can't touch your clitoris after about 20 or 30 seconds, see if you can turn the pain to pleasure by taking deep breaths and exhaling forcefully. Some women find that they can continue stimulation *through* the pain by this method, and emerge into pleasure once more.

If you still didn't have multiple orgasms, don't give up. Time is on your side. The more sex you have, the more likely you are to become multi-orgasmic. The body learns and responds by, for example, increasing the density of blood vessels in the genitals. Sexually active women naturally become more orgasmic as they get older. Interestingly, some women experience their first multiple orgasms whilst pregnant (see Chapter 12). Every week, set aside one hour for 'multiple orgasm training' and keep on until you succeed.

MULTIPLE ORGASMS WITH YOUR PARTNER

If you have a partner who only wants to orgasm once himself, as is usually the case, it may be that he assumes you only need to orgasm once as well. Quite probably, because of him, you've accepted the idea that one is enough for you too.

Once you've mastered multi-orgasms on your own, you need to let your partner know that you want to try for more with him. Don't be embarrassed about it. Some women are afraid they'll be thought of as nymphomaniacs but most men respond very positively to the idea of 'giving' their partners multiple orgasms. The more orgasms a woman has, the more macho the man feels. The more you enjoy yourself, the more he's going to enjoy himself.

The ideal is to have several orgasms before your partner has his, and then to have one 'big one' together. The majority of multi-orgasmic women say three to five is about right, but a few women have the feeling they'll never be satisfied because, with each orgasm, the drive keeps growing and growing. A few rare women have multiple orgasms that *seem* to be one continuous orgasm (only scientific instruments can make the distinction) lasting for perhaps a minute, an experience known as 'status orgasmus'.

Have a go

Depending on your partner's skill and ability to control himself, you should aim to have at least one and possibly several orgasms *before* intercourse.

► *Give yourself one orgasm with a vibrator (see Chapter 9) while your partner is in the shower.*
► *Have a second orgasm from your partner giving you oral sex.*
► *Have a third orgasm with your partner inside you, while you masturbate at the same time.*
► *Finish with simultaneous orgasms brought about by his thrusting. This may be a more profound, whole-body experience than by clitoral stimulation alone and, almost certainly, you will feel completely satisfied.*

Of course, for you to enjoy your multi-orgasmic capacity to the full it helps if your partner has good control. If he learns to become multi-orgasmic too, he'll develop that control. The next section explains how he can do this.

Multiple orgasms for men

There's been a great deal of publicity about multiple orgasms for men. What exactly are they? And are they really possible?

Having multiple orgasms doesn't mean having several of the kind of orgasm you have now. They are totally different. Multiple orgasms for men are both *less* and *more* than the normal kind.

First of all, let me try to explain in what way multiple orgasms are more than normal orgasms. You may find it hard to believe at the moment, but multiple orgasms can:

▶ *change your sex life*
▶ *change your personality*
▶ *change your relationship*
▶ *introduce a mystical element into lovemaking (it sounds crazy but it's true).*

Now let me tell you in what way multiple orgasms are less than normal orgasms. William Masters and Virginia Johnson observed one young man who ejaculated three times in ten minutes. He was a rare exception; nobody has yet found a way for the average man to ejaculate again and again in a short space of time. What are known as 'multiple orgasms' for men come at a price: you have to *forgo* ejaculation. Yes, you heard correctly. If you thought ejaculation was the whole point of sex, then prepare for a new way of thinking. No ejaculation until the last orgasm, if you so choose.

If you're puzzled by this because you think orgasm and ejaculation are one and the same thing then take a look again at Chapter 3. It's the ejaculation, not the orgasm, that brings sex to an end for most men. If you could only learn how to orgasm without the ejaculation, you could have sex indefinitely. And, in fact, you *can* learn. The technique I'm about to describe is not difficult.

First, there's something else I have to tell you. Not only do these multiple orgasms not involve ejaculation, but the orgasms themselves are somewhat unusual. Some sexologists call them 'contractile-phase orgasms' or 'pelvic orgasms' but I prefer to call them 'partial orgasms', because that's what they are.

Now that I've told you this, you may be wondering if you wouldn't prefer an ordinary old-fashioned orgasm/ejaculation after all. The idea of only having part of what you formerly had may not sound very appealing, and yet these partial orgasms can be exquisite. Once you get good at the technique, you'll find that each is more powerful than the previous one. Eventually you'll reach a state of ecstasy. Here's a list of some of the advantages of multiple orgasms:

▶ *You'll never be afraid of not being able to perform.*
▶ *You won't lose your sexual vitality in the way you do with 'ordinary' sex.*
▶ *You and your partner can have sex more often – once a day, for example, or even several times a day.*
▶ *After a session of multiple orgasms, you won't have the flat feeling you do with ejaculation.*
▶ *Your hormone balance will be different – you'll feel more affectionate and loving.*
▶ *You'll feel 'mystical'.*

Some sexologists also give these advantages:

▶ *You and your partner can enjoy sex for longer.*
▶ *Because lovemaking lasts longer, your partner will enjoy multiple orgasms as well.*

However, I wouldn't attribute these last two advantages to multiple orgasms as such. I would say that they're the result of a man learning *better control*. This improved control can be used to produce multiple orgasms but it can equally be used to achieve a longer conventional sex session.

WHAT DO MULTIPLE ORGASMS FEEL LIKE?

When you have the first of a series of multiple orgasms, you experience the beginning of a normal sequence of orgasm and ejaculation. You have that same feeling in your brain as you do when you know orgasm/ejaculation is about to happen. You have that same feeling of tensing somewhere at the base of your penis. And then ... nothing. Nothing, because the orgasm goes no further and ejaculation doesn't take place.

Put like that, it doesn't sound too great, but when you have the second orgasm, the feeling in your brain lasts fractionally longer and so does the feeling in your groin. When you have the third, the feeling is intensified again. Eventually, you reach a state in which each of these partial orgasms floods your brain with chemicals that induce an exquisite state of delirium. The initial feelings are far less than a normal orgasm/ejaculation; the ultimate feelings far surpass the normal orgasm/ejaculation.

When lovemaking is over, you don't feel sleepy, you don't feel exhausted, you don't feel depleted and yet you do feel satisfied. You also feel changed. A prolonged almost mystical state of contentment follows. You feel physically and emotionally close to your partner, and those feelings continue. If you have sex again fairly soon, this magical state of grace will never leave you.

HOW YOU CAN EXPERIENCE GREAT MULTIPLE ORGASMS

Some sexologists describe methods of physically blocking ejaculation. I don't recommend them. Some require months of training, some interfere too much with lovemaking, some are painful, some don't work and some are downright dangerous. And, in fact, there's very little to be gained by preventing the emission of semen once ejaculation has begun. Instead, I'm going to describe a very simple blend of techniques that most men will be able to master in a short time and without any risk to themselves.

Have a go
Stand naked, sideways to a full-length mirror and contract your PC muscle. You'll see that your testicles rise up closer

(Contd)

to your body. Now, let your tongue flop out of your mouth and breathe out in a series of pants. Your testicles will drop down again. That's one part of the technique for preventing ejaculation, because when you relax, and when your testicles drop away from your body, so ejaculation is less likely. Two other parts are 'Stop/Go' and the locking method already described in Chapter 3. And the most important part of all is the power of your own mind, which, as we saw in Chapter 7, is considerable. So let's put it all together.

There is one complication. There's a time delay between sensing the inevitability of ejaculation and the ejaculation actually taking place. In other words, you can cease stimulation and think you've 'got away with it', only to have ejaculation begin up to three seconds later. While you're experimenting, things are often going to 'go wrong' like this. Never mind. Enjoy it.

Before you try with your partner you'll first need to practise during masturbation. At the outset make up your mind about two things. First, you're going to masturbate for half an hour. Second, you won't ejaculate. Not during the half hour, and not at the end. Instead, when the 30 minutes is up, you'll simply stop and get on with something else.

Use Stop/Go, gradually building excitement. Once you get close to the PNR, employ the locking method. To remind you, that means contracting the PC and abdominal muscles at the same time, as if trying to crush your internal organs. That should permit you to ride right up to the PNR and then retreat again. Each time, take a little more risk until the moment you feel you've gone just that little bit too far. This is the moment to act decisively. Thrust your tongue out like a dog and pant rapidly but with much longer exhalations than inhalations. At the same instant, bring to bear all the power of your mind. Don't give in to that overwhelming desire to ejaculate. Instead:

- ▶ *stop fantasizing (if you were)*
- ▶ *stop looking at sexy images (if you were)*
- ▶ *stop 'talking dirty' (if you were)*
- ▶ *stop concentrating on the sensations.*

In other words, you have to turn off your arousal like a light.

If you've done it all correctly, instead of an ejaculation you should feel a partial orgasm, but with no semen being expelled. Don't be disappointed if your first partial orgasm is weak. Resume stimulation as soon as it's safe and the second will be better. The third better still. Eventually, you'll experience sensations that will be almost unbearably exquisite.

MULTIPLE ORGASMS WITH A PARTNER

Trying to experience multiple orgasms with a partner introduces complications. The first thing is to let her know what you're intending to do because you're going to need her co-operation. When you need to stop, it's no good if she continues to go. She has to cease stimulation as well.

In fact, the first time you try with your partner may not be hugely enjoyable for either of you. You're going to have to concentrate hard on what you're doing and that means taking attention away from her. If your partner is trying to help you, she too will be concentrating on your starting and stopping to avoid tipping you over into ejaculation. Rather than have more orgasms, she may at first have less. But don't give up after just one or two less than mind-blowing sessions; you need to give it, say, a month before you decide whether it's something you want to do regularly, occasionally, or not at all. With practice, you'll find you can control yourself with less effort and your partner will find she can once again relax into her own orgasms.

Have a go

The technique is just the same as when you were masturbating. Decide that you are not going to ejaculate. It won't work if you wait to see how you feel when the moment comes; you must be adamant in your own mind. When you get close to the level of excitement at which orgasm occurs, switch to a position that puts you in control of the movement (if you're not in one already). As soon as you start to experience a partial orgasm:

- ▶ *stop all movement*
- ▶ *stop tensing your muscles (in the locking method or otherwise)*
- ▶ *pant*
- ▶ *stop all 'dirty talk'*
- ▶ *stop all fantasizing*
- ▶ *stop looking at your partner's body*
- ▶ *stop stimulation of every kind.*

Insight

At the very moment you're about to pass the PNR you'll need to minimize the stimulation to your penis. If you stop exactly where you are, undulations along the walls of the vagina might just send you over. If you withdraw your penis completely from your partner's vagina the caress from her entrance and vaginal lips might do the same. The best option is usually to slide all the way *in*, not out, because the ballooning of the vagina just in front of the cervix means there will be no stimulation there at all.

TO EJACULATE OR NOT TO EJACULATE

The fact that you've enjoyed multiple orgasms doesn't mean that you can't ejaculate at the end of the session. If you've enjoyed only a few partial orgasms it's likely that your climactic ejaculation will be unusually powerful. On the other hand, if you've had a lot of partial orgasms during a very lengthy session you may find your ejaculation less forceful than usual. Eastern thought explains this in terms of the energy being transmitted from the pelvic area to other parts of the body. Westerners simply see it in terms of sex hormones becoming depleted and the sexual organs becoming fatigued.

Insight

You can use this 'genital fatigue' to advantage for really extended lovemaking. Every man is different but as a rule of thumb the 'danger zone' for unintended ejaculation is the first 20 minutes. If you can get beyond that you should find it possible to continue sex without ejaculation almost indefinitely.

Men who are multi-orgasmic have different ways of dealing with the question of ejaculation. Some ejaculate at the end of every session of multiple orgasms, some ejaculate at the end of sessions only occasionally, and some reserve ejaculatory sex for completely separate sessions.

What will you do? When you do ejaculate you'll lose several of the advantages of the technique. On the other hand, if you don't ejaculate your partner may feel something vital is missing. And if you've thought of simultaneous orgasm as the pinnacle of sex, then you're both going to miss it.

YOUR PARTNER'S PERSPECTIVE

Funnily enough, the greatest problem many couples have with multiple orgasms for men is not the man forgoing ejaculation for himself but the woman being disappointed. It can make a woman feel inadequate, in the same way that a man may feel inadequate if he fails to make his partner orgasm. The woman may feel that the man is holding back and not really making love to her at all. Something may seem to be lacking in the whole experience. So it's very important for you, the man, to reassure your partner about the increased pleasure she is giving you when you share this style of sex.

SO WHEN DO YOU STOP?

A man who is multi-orgasmic is on the same footing as a woman. In theory, you could both go on having sex for hours. No longer is the session brought to an end by the man's refractory period.

So how do you decide when to stop? In reality, of course, your 'sexual bodies' are going to get tired. The clitoris is going to feel numb, the vagina sore, the penis less than steel. The man is probably going to be the last to suggest stopping. Men are too competitive for that. So it's up to the woman and that's going to make her feel like a killjoy. Which is a shame. So, guys, be a bit sensitive about this. When you see that she's beginning to flag suggest that you'd find it a good moment to halt intercourse and move on to cuddles. And make it clear that you feel completely satisfied – which you almost certainly will. Most men find that a string of partial orgasms is far better than one ejaculation.

MULTI-ORGASMIC SEX AND TANTRA

Nowadays, non-ejaculation has become synonymous with what people are calling 'tantric sex', meaning that the man keeps going as long as possible so his partner can enjoy numerous orgasms. But in reality, the ritual sex that formed just a tiny part of Tantra never was about specific techniques. It was about spirituality. That was what defined it. And, in fact, the most ancient rituals centred on the 'magical power' of sexual fluids, rather than the sex itself. Nevertheless, it's true that to reach the heights of ecstasy that some Tantrikas later sought through sex does require prolonged sex sessions. And that requires a man to be multi-orgasmic (to build the state of bliss) and to be able to forgo ejaculation. But if you really want to follow the path of tantric sex, remember that the physical techniques are only a means to an end, not the end itself.

Unfortunately, there hasn't yet been enough research into what exactly happens hormonally when a man enjoys multi-orgasmic sex. But from my own observations the results are very positive. Whether or not you consider yourself to be a spiritual person, and whether or not you follow any religion, I would go so far as to say that introducing non-ejaculatory sessions could make you a calmer, more tranquil, less irritable person and enormously improve your relationship.

10 THINGS TO REMEMBER

1 Most women can become multi-orgasmic.

2 Masturbation is the best way for women to learn to become multi-orgasmic.

3 Women who aren't multi-orgasmic may not have a positive enough attitude to masturbation.

4 Women who have sex regularly automatically become more multi-orgasmic.

5 Multiple orgasms for men are really a series of partial orgasms without ejaculation.

6 At first, male multiple orgasms may not feel very exciting but as skill improves they can induce a state of delirium far beyond a conventional orgasm/ejaculation.

7 The locking method is the best way of delaying ejaculation.

8 Panting and mental control are the keys to halting an impending ejaculation and thus achieving multiple orgasms for men.

9 Have sessions of intercourse in which you both enjoy only multiple orgasms and have completely separate sessions when you enjoy simultaneous orgasm together, with the man ejaculating.

10 Multiple orgasms and non-ejaculation are among the techniques that can be used to achieve a spiritual state in Tantra.

HOW GREAT IS SEX NOW?

▶ *Have you practised having multiple orgasms during masturbation?*   Yes/No

▶ *Women: if you haven't been able to experience multiple orgasms, have you really run through all the suggestions without inhibition?*   Yes/No

▶ *Men: have you masturbated for half an hour without ejaculating?*   Yes/No

▶ *Men: if you haven't yet achieved non-ejaculatory masturbation, have you really tried all the techniques with a firm resolve?*   Yes/No

▶ *Have you been able to achieve multiple orgasms during sex?*   Yes/No

▶ *Have you been able to help your partner achieve multiple orgasms during sex?*   Yes/No

▶ *Men: have you been able to have intercourse without ejaculating?*   Yes/No

▶ *Have you found a way of bringing non-ejaculatory sessions to an end without anybody's feelings being hurt?*   Yes/No

▶ *Have you found that multiple orgasms have made you feel more spiritual?*   Yes/No

If you answered 'no' to more than three questions, re-read the relevant parts of the chapter and make an effort to put the suggestions into effect. If you're a woman and having problems becoming multi-orgasmic, don't get frustrated about it. Time is on your side. Enjoy practising and it will happen one day. Guys, time is also on your side when it comes to controlling ejaculation – it becomes easier as you get older. Don't forget that both of you will need to make psychological adjustments once you've developed the ability to enjoy sex without ejaculating. Women may miss the simultaneous fireworks you used to enjoy together. The answer is to alternate between non-ejaculatory sex sessions and ejaculatory sessions.

9

Great toys, tricks and aphrodisiacs

In this chapter you will learn:
- *how sex toys can enhance your experience*
- *special techniques to use occasionally*
- *safe aphrodisiacs that really work.*

Without doubt, great sex can be entirely 'natural'. However, we live in the twenty-first century. In every other aspect of human experience we expect progress, so why not in sex? Technology has brought new and more powerful ways of creating stimulation and I suggest you try them out. If you don't like them there's no harm done. But the chances are that you'll like quite a few of them, at least for occasional use.

Sex toys

If you're bold enough, make a trip to your nearest sex shop to take a look. You'll find a huge range of sex toys there. Ideally, go as a couple and make it a bit of an occasion. Fight the impulse to turn and flee the moment you step through the door. Some things will surprise you, some will make you laugh, some will probably evoke a 'yuk', and some you may end up buying. If there isn't a sex shop near you, or you're too embarrassed to go in, take a look on the internet.

VIBRATORS

The standard sex toy is the vibrator. If you haven't got one, get one. They sell in their millions and there's absolutely nothing 'kinky' about them at all. Women use them on their own, men use them on their own, and couples use them together.

The traditional vibrator is approximately the size and shape of a penis, either in a realistic skin colour or in anything from white to fluorescent orange. More recently other designs have been introduced because, in fact, most women prefer the vibrations on or close to the clitoris, not in the vagina and don't therefore need the penis shape.

Other innovations include protrusions for stimulating the clitoris while the main barrel is inside the vagina, and designs in which the 'penis' not only vibrates but also rotates. Yet another category can be worn by a woman against her clitoris, with the vibrator incorporated into a G-string. You can get vibrators that attach to mobile phones – so you're always pleased when your partner phones – and even to your iPod, to give you orgasms in time to music.

Vibrators aren't generally very expensive so, over a period of time, you can experiment with different designs. If you're buying your first, it's probably best to go for a standard penis shape. You'll have to decide between soft and hard models. Most people opt for soft vibrators, initially, because they seem more friendly but, in fact, it's the hard designs that deliver the most intense vibrations. For the maximum stimulation, buy a mains powered model. Some vibrators have large heads the size of a ping-pong ball and are marketed as body massagers. When applied to the pelvic area, the vibrations are spectacular and deep but they also tend to be diffused so it's worth paying a little extra for a detachable head that can, when needed, concentrate the sensations on the clitoris, G-spot or penis. Be warned that some women – and men – find mains powered models so powerful that they actually go numb.

How do you use a vibrator? Men buy them to excite their partners and immediately set about plunging them in and out. Not many women appreciate this. The most effective technique is to apply the tip of the vibrator on or close to the clitoris, depending on how sensitive the woman is, and to keep it *still*. In fact, it's usually better for the woman to do this for herself. A vibrator is a great toy for a woman to masturbate alone.

If you've never considered a vibrator, you may be asking: 'What on earth's the point?' The answer (apart from variety) is that, in general, women take a little longer than men to become aroused. The vibrator allows them to, as it were, catch up. Of course, it's just one way but it's a good one. Don't forget that vibrators can also be used on men; this can be just for fun or to help when a man has erection problems. Simply press against the penis. For men there are also artificial vaginas with a very realistic natural skin feel.

Women who have never had an orgasm often experience their first one with a vibrator. The less orgasmic a woman is, the more powerful the vibrator needs to be. If you don't orgasm easily, you'll almost certainly find that you can 'train' yourself quite quickly. In one of my focus groups, a woman in her thirties told me how she'd never had an orgasm with any man (a problem known as 'situational anorgasmia') until she began using a vibrator and, within a month, became multi-orgasmic during intercourse.

When you're together as a couple, the woman can masturbate with the vibrator for her own pleasure and your entertainment, building up the initial excitement (and lubrication). Later, the vibrator can provide additional stimulation in a position where it's difficult to reach the clitoris. For example, when she's lying flat on the bed, face down, the vibrator can be slipped underneath, against her vulva.

Some vibrators are designed specifically for the G-spot. These models have a tip that's curved or even at right-angles to the body. Again, it's far easier for the woman to find the right spot herself than for her partner to do it (because he won't be getting any direct feedback as he would with his finger). Many women, however, say that it's pressure on the G-spot, rather than vibration, that works the magic. These women prefer a dildo.

DILDOS

Dildos have been in use for thousands of years. You could say
they're vibrators without vibrations. The latest generation is
made of glass (usually pyrex). Whereas vibrators are made of
various kinds of plastic and find it hard to escape a tacky image,
many of these glass dildos are extremely elegant. Some even come
with stands so they can be displayed beside the bed. Glass has
particular qualities. It can be put in the fridge for a cool sensation,
or into a mug of warm water. Being incredibly smooth, little or
no lubrication is required. And being non-porous, glass is very
hygienic – a glass dildo can even be put in the dishwasher.

If you like the idea of glass but also want vibrations, there are
models that have a hole into which a vibrating 'bullet' can be
inserted – or you can simply touch a vibrator to the end. Glass
transmits the vibrations extremely well, which gives you the best
of both worlds.

ANAL TOYS

The anus is a highly erogenous area in both men and women,
and there are vibrators specially designed for it. They're usually
narrower than standard models. Some have a wide base so they
can't accidentally slip all the way in. An exciting way of using
an anal vibrator is to slide it into the woman's rectum during
intercourse, so you can both feel the sensations. A man can also
insert one into his rectum during intercourse, to intensify his
own stimulation.

Double vibrators come in two sorts. One kind has the 'penises' side
by side for simultaneous vaginal and anal penetration. Another
kind has them pointing in opposite directions. These are aimed
principally at lesbians, but heterosexual couples can also use them,
the woman having one end in her vagina while the man has the
other in his anus.

Harnesses and strap-ons exist that will allow a woman to act the
part of a man. Again these can be used by lesbians but also by
heterosexual couples who want to switch roles. The man can feel
what it's like to be penetrated (in the rectum), and the woman can
feel what it's like to do the penetrating.

There are also dildos for the anal canal and rectum. The simplest
are known as 'butt plugs' and they stretch the ring of muscle for an
'open' sensation. For women they additionally give a fuller, tighter
feeling during vaginal intercourse and can also relax the sphincter
for anal intercourse afterwards. For men, there are very special
models precisely designed to massage the prostate. Women can use
them on men or men can use them on themselves – rhythmically
flexing the PC muscle causes the tip of the toy to do its work.

OTHER SEX TOYS

Vibrating 'cock rings' are worn around the base of the penis.
The man feels the vibrations along his penis and, as a result, the
woman feels them inside her vagina. In addition, some of these
toys are designed to press on the clitoris. The earlier models were
rather cumbersome with wires that got in the way, but there's now

a new generation of throwaway rings powered by a tiny built-in battery.

A word of caution about cock rings that actually constrict the penis. They're supposed to help a man keep an erection by stopping the blood from flowing out but they *can do damage*. Never take any risks with your penis.

Other kinds of sex toys that you might like to try include love balls that clunk around inside the vagina (and can be kept in during intercourse), nipple vibrators, and inflatable cushions specially designed for those more difficult positions.

Bondage

There's a whole psychology based around bondage. It can sound very alarming, but it isn't at all. Bondage itself has nothing to do with inflicting pain. It's basically an extreme expression of the basic concept that women like to have things done to them and men like to do those things. When tied down to a bed, for example, a woman is no longer responsible for anything that happens. She is, in effect, absolved of guilt, and that can be very important to some women.

Men, too, sometimes enjoy being tied up or, rather, the things a woman might do while they're tied up. It can be a tantalizing and beautiful 'torture'. A woman can perform a striptease, masturbate, bring her body close but not close enough to touch, arouse him a little, then go away leaving him in a state of delicious anticipation.

A whole range of bondage accessories is available in sex shops or on the internet but, to start with, you can use things that are to hand.

It's normally the man who wants to introduce the idea of bondage, and it's not an easy thing to tell a partner. (If it's the woman who's curious, on the other hand, then her partner is unlikely to object.) You could try introducing the subject when you're fantasizing together (see Chapter 7). Or you could say that you'd like her to tie you up. Once you've had some fun with that, she may be open to reversing roles.

In fact, some women are just as excited by the idea of bondage as some men are but they're also likely to be suspicious. Your partner will be wondering why you want to do it. After all, restricting a woman's movements doesn't sound like a recipe for great sex.

A woman is right to be cautious. Never allow yourself to be tied up by a man you don't know *extremely* well. Even someone you've been with quite a while may reveal a side to his character you never dreamed of. I would advise you not to permit any restraints initially that can't, if necessary, be undone or broken by you. If you both enjoy yourselves and all is well, you can move on to something stronger later on.

There are some things that you can do that have a whiff of bondage about them without the woman actually being restrained. For example, in a missionary position you could raise your partner's hands above her head and hold them there (in other words, her arms are stretched out along the pillow or bed behind her). You could, when undressing her in bed, pull her underwear down to her knees or ankles and leave it there. If she's agreeable and flexible enough, with her underwear around her knees she could pull her legs back and you could slip the gusset behind her head. If she's less flexible (or has flimsy underwear), you can achieve the same effect with a scarf.

Handcuffs are quite popular. To begin with, use cheap plastic ones that can be broken easily. Only use metal ones if you're totally confident. Either of you could have your arms handcuffed behind your back, for example. For a laugh, you could both wear handcuffs and see if you can manage to make love at all.

The next level is for one of you to be tied spread-eagled to the bed. Of course, you need to have a suitable bed. But being tied up is only the start. The person who isn't tied up still has to *do* something.

If you're the person who's free, give your partner your full
attention without thinking about your own satisfaction. This is
the one time your partner can just lie back and enjoy it, but you
have to be as inventive as possible. Surprise your partner – but
make sure it's a nice surprise. Try stimulating your partner's skin
with different things – feathers, a brush, ice, massage oil, whatever
you can think of. Take a look at some of the ideas below and see
how you might incorporate them into a bondage session. Push the
boundaries further than they've been pushed before – but only a
little further.

Bondage often goes hand in hand with a certain style of dressing up
for sex. Rubber dresses and underwear are popular. Many women
who aren't interested in bondage nevertheless find this 'dominatrix'
style attractive and arousing.

Pain and pleasure

They don't call it slap and tickle for nothing. The fact is that
a little bit of physical pain increases sexual arousal. No doubt
there's a connection with the sexual habits of our less sophisticated
relatives – in mammals, many males bite the females while
having sex, especially around the neck. Hence love bites. In fact,
the hormonal response to stress is very similar to the hormonal
response in sexual arousal.

However, I'm not for a moment suggesting that *real pain* should
be involved. I'm talking about just enough sensation to increase
vasocongestion.

Insight

Men, but also women, sometimes spontaneously smack their partners on the buttocks during the excitement of sex. The fact is that the smacking causes blood to rush to the area, augmenting the arousal of the pelvic organs. Men often fantasize about spanking women and women sometimes fantasize about being spanked. That's something you can, now and then, incorporate into love play if you both agree.

The question is, how much pain equals pleasure, and how much is too much? The first step is to try things out on yourself while masturbating. Try pinching, biting, scratching, spanking and pulling tufts of pubic hair. Generally, the more aroused you are, the more the sensation of pain is perceived as pleasure.

There are other ways of increasing stress hormones in the blood (although not necessarily vasocongestion). For example, there's stress. Things like a fairground ride, or, at the high end of the scale, a parachute jump. And around the house and garden, there's always a good old chasing game.

Insight

Ice applied to the nipples can cause spectacular erection. A handful shoved unexpectedly into the underwear tends to liven things up a bit. Some women report that an ice cube slipped into the vagina just before sex leads to an arousing trickle on the inner thighs while others claim it's best just before climax.

Role-playing

In the late-Victorian period an Austrian academic wrote a short book about a man who, to demonstrate his love, offered to become his mistress's servant. The book was called *Venus In Furs* and the author, who based the story on his own life, was called Leopold von Sacher-Masoch. Although the story did end in humiliation and pain, giving the word 'masochism' to the world, it was more than anything else a tale of role-playing. Nowadays there are couples who call themselves masochists who do nothing more than act out little scenarios in which one agrees (up to a point) to do whatever the other wishes. For a time, one is dominant, the other subservient. Sometimes 'contracts' are signed covering a day, a weekend or longer. Probably not many couples will want to follow this route but for those who are particularly inhibited, role-playing can be valuable. For example, by agreeing to perform any sexual act your partner desires, you become absolved of any responsibility yourself. In that way, you can experience something you had really wanted to do but had been afraid to ask for. And, in a few hours you'll probably get to know more about your partner's inner world than you would have found out in years.

Insight

Of course, everyone has a limit in role-playing. Hopefully, your partner would understand yours without being asked but, just to be on the safe side, you should always agree that the scenario can be brought to an end at any time. Decide on a code word for 'no' beforehand otherwise your partner won't know if you really want to stop or if your protestations are just part of your role-play.

Lubrication

I've mentioned lubrication before and I'm going to mention it again, because it's very important, especially for older couples. Saliva is a standard lubricant. It's effective, it's about the right viscosity, it's readily available and it's free, but there are better ones. Some are available in the chemist, but for a wide selection you'll have to go to a sex shop or buy on the internet (see 'Taking it further' for addresses). There's a huge variety available now. The latest generation contains silicone, and their advantage is that they're very long lasting and extremely slippery. Curiously, they don't actually feel wet and some couples find they don't enhance pleasure in the way more conventional lubricants do. With non-silicone lubricants, be ready to 'top up' several times during long sessions.

Remember that only silicone and water-based lubricants should be used with latex condoms. Oil-based lubricants can make holes in the latex.

Insight

If you're using condoms, try 'gel charging' as a way of enhancing male pleasure. While the condom is still rolled up, fill the 'teat' at the end with water-based lubricant, then put on the condom as usual. During intercourse, the lubricant floods out from the tip of the condom to produce an intense sensation of wetness. Some men like it so much they wear a condom even if they have no reason to.

Don't forget you can lubricate all of your body, not just your genitals. Something that feels wet and slippery on your skin definitely enhances the sensation of touch.

Insight

Because they're so slippery, silicone lubricants can be used to prolong sex. Just apply more than you normally would and the reduced friction will make it easier for a man to keep going without ejaculating.

Aphrodisiacs

An aphrodisiac is something that excites sexual desire but I also use the term to mean something that improves sexual performance. There's no doubt that when you feel sexually charged up, you naturally feel more desire.

The most important aphrodisiac is sex itself. When you have sex frequently, both your body and your mind come to expect it and miss it when it doesn't happen. If, for some reason, your partner has gone off sex, see if you can't gently persuade him or her to at least try frequent sex for a while. Even if your partner only agrees reluctantly, it may be the case that a few sessions will be enough to kickstart hormone production. If not, you may be tempted to try hormone supplements. After all, it seems fairly straightforward. If a certain hormone promotes sexual desire or performance, then why not take a substance that either contains the hormone or helps create it? The problem is that the body is constantly changing one chemical into another chemical. You can't be sure the chemical you put in won't end up as a completely different chemical. Testosterone, the 'male' hormone, is a good example. As a supplement it can, in some cases, actually end up by increasing levels of oestrogen, the 'female' hormone. Not what you wanted.

When you use pills and potions, you also have to consider the possible side effects. I would strongly recommend that you do not experiment recreationally with 'prescription' drugs such as Viagra and Cialis. If you don't have an erection problem, you don't need anything this powerful. If you do have an erection problem, you should see a doctor and let the doctor decide what treatment is appropriate. These kinds of drugs have side effects which, in certain cases, can be severe. In addition, if you buy on the internet, it's difficult to be sure what you're actually getting.

There are various 'natural' aphrodisiacs and performance boosters but, for most of them their immediate and long-term effects have not been properly studied. The problem with this area of research is the so-called 'placebo effect'. If you think you're being given an aphrodisiac, you tend to get excited at the very idea of it. In one test, for example, 10 per cent of men given a placebo for sexual dysfunction showed an improvement. Women seem to be even more susceptible: in a study of 77 women, 42 per cent reported increased sexual desire, 35 per cent said they had more clitoral sensation, and 30 per cent said they had more frequent orgasms after taking a placebo. As I pointed out in Chapter 7, the power of the mind should never be underestimated.

This is not to say that natural products don't work, of course. In that same study on women, the real product being tested (a mixture of L-arginine, Panax ginseng, Ginkgo biloba, Damiana and various vitamins and minerals) scored considerably higher than the placebo in all categories. Nevertheless, you can see that when claims are made without a properly designed scientific study, the placebo effect may significantly distort the findings. What's more, natural substances that are known to have at least some real effect can have serious side effects. That applies, for example, to Yohimbe and Ephedra.

From personal experience, there are certain herbs that I'm convinced do work. However, I can't rule out the placebo effect on myself, nor is it worth taking risks over side effects if you don't actually have anything wrong with you. If you're over 50, take a look at Chapter 13 and if you're suffering from serious erectile dysfunction take a look at Chapter 14, but otherwise my advice is that you and your partner work on your bodies from the 'inside'.

I explain how you can do that in Chapter 11. Meanwhile, as you now see, there are many aphrodisiacs other than pills that can have a safe and powerful effect.

> **Warning:** Never secretly slip an 'aphrodisiac' into your partner's food or drink. That would be a gross violation of human rights, apart from which he or she may be taking medication or have a medical condition that makes the substance dangerous.

STRIPTEASE, LINGERIE AND MORE

There can hardly be a man on the planet who doesn't respond to striptease, yet it's not an easy thing for most women to do. For information on where to get lessons in all that bumping and grinding take a look at 'Taking it further'.

You also need the right kind of underwear. Most men are turned on by lingerie. In particular, fishnet stockings, suspender belts and corsets. It's partly a question of the kinds of images seen in men's magazines and partly a question of the way garments can emphasize a woman's shape and frame her most exciting features.

Be inventive. Don't stick with the standard 'outfit' every time. Quite a lot of men find a pair of high-heeled boots complement a corset very well. Keep them on to make love. They also look rather well on a woman wearing cowboy chaps and a cowboy hat and nothing else. Or what about a choker worn with elbow-length gloves? Or a raincoat with nothing underneath?

The idea of ripping clothes off appeals to many men. So don't throw your old clothes away; keep them for a session of some really ripping fun.

SHAVING AND WAXING

Although some men prefer hairy women (and it's true that the hair traps vaginal scent), the consensus seems to be that a clear view of the vulva is enormously exciting to a man, especially the first time. Try surprising your man. Or let him trim your locks to his own personal taste as a little bit of love play.

There are various ways of going about things. If you use an electric razor make sure it's designed for the purpose – a man's beard trimmer can nick folds of flesh. For a really smooth job, many women nowadays prefer a professional waxing, although the stubble will return after a week or so. An economical solution favoured by many women is to regularly use a disposable razor and shave against the grain, using shaving cream or soap. (The first time you'll have to cut the hair short, very carefully, with scissors.)

The general idea is to remove all the hair from around the outer vaginal lips, leaving just a little tuft on the mons. If you have fairly extensive hair on the mons, you may be able to do something interesting with it, like trim it into a V-shape. Some women remove everything.

Apart from making your man very excited indeed, you'll find the sensitivity of your genital area considerably increased.

Guys, there probably isn't much point in trying to excite your partner by fully exposing your penis and testicles. Most women aren't very interested. However, a cunning use of your partner's electric razor can make your penis look longer, which can be good for confidence, as well as making fellatio more agreeable for her. As with a woman, shaving bare may also increase sensitivity – a lubricated hand gliding over smooth skin can be extremely sensual.

EROTICA

It's always been said that women are more turned on by the written word while men are excited by visual images. Yet the culture is changing. In my focus groups, increasing numbers of women admit to being aroused by erotic films.

By the way, the dictionary doesn't make a distinction between the words 'erotic' and 'pornographic', but many people, and some feminists in particular, do use the words differently. Essentially, 'erotic' has become a positive word while 'pornographic' has become negative, especially in the sense of showing scenes in which women are exploited and degraded. Here, I talk about films that are erotic.

For a start, why not take turns reading some erotica out loud to one another? You'll get turned on and you'll maybe try to copy what you've been reading. At the very least, it should provoke some interesting discussion.

If that goes well, try an erotic film. I often hear people say sex films are 'boring'. Well, it all depends in what frame of mind you view them. It's a little bit like laughter. If you're not willing to laugh, the funniest comedian in the world will leave you unmoved. When you feel in the mood to laugh, the most trivial joke can have you in hysterics.

With a sex film, the director doesn't expect you to *watch* it from start to finish. He or she expects you to be rolling about on the floor, either on your own or with your partner. Those interminable scenes are there for you to masturbate to or make love to. If they only lasted a few seconds, you wouldn't have time for either.

It's a fact that every normal person is excited by seeing images of other people having sex, whether they admit it or not. But it's equally true that different people react very differently to the same scene.

Women tend to like to see lovemaking from a little distance. Men tend to like the camera to be right up close. Consequently, it's difficult to find erotic films that will appeal equally to both of you. You probably won't find anything suitable among the hardcore titles in your sex shop. Look instead in your local rental outlet or search for 'couple friendly films' on the internet (see 'Taking it further' for addresses). Incidentally, you can't buy hardcore (R18) films by mail order in the UK, only those with an 18 certificate.

Insight

If you've got your partner tied up, as described above, it could be a good moment to put on an erotic film, especially if he or she has never seen one before.

MIRRORS AND CAMERAS

Quite apart from being excited by images of other people making love, just about everyone gets excited by images of themselves making love. The easiest way to experiment with this is to use a mirror. If you have one on a stand, bring it up by the bed. The best is probably a mirror on the wall behind the bed, angled slightly downwards.

With cameras, a large part of the excitement is simply in the idea of them. It's partly the satisfaction of curiosity and partly the frisson of being 'watched', even if it is only by a machine.

In the old days, you had to use a Polaroid-type camera to get an instant result (and avoid sending film to a processing laboratory), but nowadays there are digital cameras. Better still there are camcorders. Women with an exhibitionist tendency tend to find the notion pretty exciting, but get worried about the idea of the images falling into somebody else's hands. A word of warning, girls. Don't do it if you're not 100 per cent sure of your partner. If he were to try to sell the images, or just circulate them among his friends, he wouldn't be the first. If you find the idea a turn-on but are a little worried, insist on having the flash memory, cassette or whatever. Most of the fun, anyway, is in the filming rather than the watching. You can enjoy both simultaneously if you link your camcorder up to your TV to watch yourselves in real time (and you don't have to record it if you don't want to).

APHRODISIACS FOR WOMEN

Many women are aroused by the aphrodisiacs described here (as well as in Chapters 4 and 7), but there's no doubt that women are far more individual than men in this respect. In my focus groups, women have spoken about things as varied as the scent of their partners' bodies, the sight of the muscles on their arms, and a few words of appreciation and praise as being enough to do the trick. For many women with 'insufficient libido', their partners may find that attention to such things as personal hygiene and the development of genuine empathy are all the aphrodisiacs that are necessary.

10 THINGS TO REMEMBER

1 *Technology is entering most areas of life, so why not sex?*

2 *Shop together for sex toys – either in a sex shop or online.*

3 *At the very least, every couple should have a vibrator.*

4 *Bondage can be an opportunity for one of you to really lie back and enjoy it.*

5 *A slap (not too hard) along with the tickle heightens arousal.*

6 *Role-playing can be a way of overcoming inhibitions.*

7 *Lubrication is vital for great sex.*

8 *Don't use pills and potions recreationally – they can have dangerous side effects.*

9 *Good aphrodisiacs for men include lingerie and a shaven or waxed vulva.*

10 *Good aphrodisiacs for couples include erotic books and films, mirrors and cameras.*

HOW GREAT IS SEX NOW?

▶ *Have you shopped for sex toys together?*   Yes/No

▶ *Have you, at the very least, bought and tried out a vibrator?*   Yes/No

▶ *Have you had a go at bondage?*   Yes/No

▶ *Have you tried a little 'slap' along with the 'tickle'?*   Yes/No

▶ *Have you experimented with artificial lubricants?*   Yes/No

▶ *Have you practised some striptease and given your partner a performance?*   Yes/No

▶ *Have you watched an erotic film together?*   Yes/No

▶ *Have you watched yourselves making love in a mirror or by using some sort of video recorder?*   Yes/No

If you answered 'no' to more than three questions, re-read the relevant parts of the chapter and make an effort to put the suggestions into effect. It's important to open yourselves up to new ideas and the possibilities offered by new technology, so you always have something to look forward to that you've never tried before. There's nothing 'kinky' about anything in this chapter. Vibrators sell in their millions. Most of the time you may prefer doing things the 'natural' way but, on occasion, new ideas can add excitement and freshness.

10

After orgasm

In this chapter you will learn:
* *why the post-orgasm period is vital to satisfaction*
* *how men are victims of their hormones*
* *why multiple orgasms for men can prolong happiness.*

The last orgasm is definitely not the end of sex. It's merely the end of an act in the whole drama of making love. The experience won't be complete unless you now revel together in the sensations you've shared.

The first seconds and minutes

Women always seem to need longer than men to descend from a sexual high (unless the man has been multi-orgasmic and not ejaculated). In fact, it takes about an hour for a woman's brain wave pattern to return to 'normal'. Therefore, the post-orgasm period is especially important to a woman; her partner should remember that.

A man should not withdraw immediately (unless he's wearing a condom). To a woman withdrawal can feel like an abandonment. Moreover, a woman can still enjoy certain gentle sensations while the penis is inside her. It's better to let the penis 'fall out' of its own accord.

Men display a variety of reactions immediately after ejaculating. The standard one is to fall asleep. Nevertheless, a man certainly shouldn't give in to the urge unless his partner wants to as well. In that case, the two of you should sleep in one another's arms.

A second reaction is for a man to want to lie awake, but on his own. If this happens with you, then there's almost certainly something wrong with the relationship.

A third reaction is for the man to become quite alert. Byron, the famous poet and womanizer, was reputed to jump out of bed and have a sword fight with the curtains.

The man's reaction depends very much on his hormone levels before sex and what happens to them during and after sex. There is an evolutionary driven mechanism at work, as you'll see below, that deliberately sets out to destroy your post-coital paradise. You have to use every technique you can to combat it.

What can be done to co-ordinate a man's descent from the high with that of his partner? Music can play a very important role. It acts on the same parts of the brain that sex does; it inhibits activity in the amygdala, which is associated with negative emotions, and stimulates reward structures such as the ventral tegmental area. In other words, the right music will help prolong that feeling of bliss.

It's nice to share a drink (perhaps from the same glass) and have some little things to eat, such as nuts or fruits (all prepared and brought into the bedroom beforehand). You can still do sexy things such as 'kiss' your drink from one to the other. (Remember that, as described in Chapter 7, a *little* alcohol *after* sex can prolong your dopamine 'hit'.)

The man should continue to be present for his partner. Try some of the cuddling positions described in Chapter 4. You should spend maybe half an hour lying together like this. While you do, reaffirm your appreciation and love for one another.

Making love should be a beautiful experience and you should aim to prolong that beautiful world for as long as possible.

The sexual hangover

Unfortunately, your private beautiful world of lovemaking doesn't necessarily suit evolution. You see, once a man and a woman have had sex and, in theory anyway, spread their genes, the survival of the species is best served if the man finds another mate. What it means in practice is that a woman who was the most beautiful being on earth just before sex, suddenly becomes one of the least desirable. This is known as the 'Coolidge Effect' and it has been very carefully studied in rats. After an orgy of sex with a particular female, a male rat will eventually lose all interest in her. In fact, he'll apparently be quite incapable of any more. And, yet, introduce a new female and, suddenly, he's able to do it again. This has been observed in female rats, too, and in many species, including, I'm afraid, humans. In my focus groups, several men have told me how they've experienced the effect for themselves, having sex with more than one partner in one night.

What exactly is going on? Dopamine has a lot to do with it. Having sex raises dopamine levels enormously, and makes men and women feel good. It's the reward for perpetuating the species. Yet after sex, dopamine levels drop sharply. Since there's no point in rewarding more sex with the same partner (who might already be pregnant), dopamine stubbornly refuses to soar again unless a new partner comes along.

This is the same mechanism that is at work in men and women whose relationships never last more than a few weeks. They're dopamine addicts, and a new partner is an easier fix than working to improve the relationship and the sex life with the existing partner. (So now you know why such men are called *rats* rather than, say, porcupines.)

This dopamine desert is all part of what's known as the 'sexual hangover', which involves a lot of other chemicals as well. A drug-induced high is always followed by a low and, unfortunately, highs produced by the body itself are not immune to this universal law. Another part of the hangover in men is a significant reduction in androgen (the male hormone) receptor density, which may take several days to return to normal. In the meantime, a man may feel less like sex and his mood will change for the worse.

In fact, not everyone necessarily looks to sex for the next dopamine high. Some find it in things like food, gambling, other kinds of risk taking, and in alcohol.

Is there anything that can be done about it? Yes, there is.

DON'T BE A SLAVE TO YOUR HORMONES

You probably never realized you were suffering from a sexual hangover. But when you roll away from your partner and wonder why on earth you had been so eager to have sex, that's the beginning of the sexual hangover. When your partner suddenly seems less beautiful or handsome, that's the sexual hangover. When she or he suddenly seems less successful and desirable, that's the sexual hangover. When the house suddenly seems dusty or the garden overgrown, that's the sexual hangover. It's all to do with your perceptions. Your hormones are urging you to pick a fight; to seek a new mate.

You don't have to give in to your hormones. And, in fact, by not giving in your body will adapt all the more quickly. It naturally seeks *homeostasis* or balance. In seeking to counterbalance the high it may create a low, but it will get the situation right, and fairly quickly, provided you don't do anything else to exacerbate the situation. While these changes are going on, try not to let them affect you too much. Use your intelligence and your powers of reasoning to try to overcome your hormones.

THE OXYTOCIN EFFECT

At some point in human development, the evolutionary tendency to favour the spreading of genes as widely as possible was counterbalanced by a new imperative. If children were to survive (and become parents in their turn) they needed to be protected. And, given their slow rate of development, that protection had to continue for years. Mum, Dad and the kids all had to bond. One of the chemicals involved in that bonding is 'oxytocin'.

Oxytocin is a wonderful hormone. It provokes uterine contractions for childbirth, it's released in the mother when a baby is breast-fed and it's released when the baby cries. It binds mother and child together. It reduces cravings, induces calm, speeds recovery from illness, increases longevity, and helps prevent impotence.

Oxytocin is also the key to monogamy. When oxytocin was injected into the brains of various promiscuous rodents, they preferred their regular partner to a new one. In other words, oxytocin is the cure for the Coolidge Effect and the sexual hangover.

So, how can you get more of this wonderful stuff? It's released during sex. In women, high levels lead to multiple orgasms (no surprise, given its role in provoking contractions of the uterus when giving birth). In men, its levels rise during sex – but following ejaculation it eventually falls to what might be called its background level.

One thing men can do is to follow an approach to life and relationships that favours oxytocin. This means lots of skin contact, lots of cuddling and lots of reflection on your partner's many wonderful qualities.

Insight

It seems that while women's oxytocin levels are higher *throughout* sex, men's peak just *prior* to orgasm. This means that by having multiple orgasms, men can build up their all-important oxytocin level.

The other thing that men can do is to stop ejaculating. There are two styles of sex in which men don't ejaculate. The first is multi-orgasmic sex, which we looked at in Chapter 8. This is a complicated area of research because some men will have only one or two weak orgasms, while other men may experience a dozen powerful ones; some men will leak a small quantity of liquid, others a larger quantity. In some cases, that liquid may contain prostatic fluid, seminal fluid and sperm; in other cases, it might involve only prostatic fluid.

The second style of sex is neither to ejaculate nor orgasm. I'm not going to say more about it now because I deal with it in Chapter 13.

What does seem clear is that when men don't ejaculate, they're left with a relatively level feeling of wellbeing and calm. Somehow the oxytocin level is high and remains high. Their partners always look beautiful.

10 THINGS TO REMEMBER

1 *The time together after the last orgasm should be just as beautiful as everything else to do with sex.*

2 *Women generally take longer than men to descend from the sexual high.*

3 *A good way of co-ordinating a man's descent with that of his partner is to cuddle while listening to romantic music together.*

4 *The Coolidge Effect means that men tend to find their partners less attractive after sex and may even think of chasing other women.*

5 *The Coolidge Effect is part of the sexual hangover, which is basically the low that follows the high of sex.*

6 *Your after-sex dopamine level can be kept up by sharing a small glass of wine.*

7 *Don't give in to your hormones when they're being negative.*

8 *Oxytocin is the key to monogamy.*

9 *Keeping oxytocin levels up helps combat the sexual hangover in men.*

10 *Sex without ejaculation keeps oxytocin levels high.*

HOW GREAT IS SEX NOW?

▶ Have you prolonged the state of after-sex bliss by
  cuddling to romantic music?   Yes/No

▶ Have you shared a small glass of wine together after
  sex (not before)?   Yes/No

▶ Are you keeping up your oxytocin levels with lots of
  skin contact and cuddles?   Yes/No

▶ If your after-sex hormones have turned negative, have
  you used the power of your mind to overcome them?   Yes/No

If you answered 'no' to more than two questions, re-read the
relevant parts of the chapter and make an effort to put the
suggestions into effect. The period after the last orgasm is just as
important as everything else in sex, especially for women. Don't
rush it. Remember that great sex is as much about the mind as the
body, and the mind can keep going long after the genitals have
given up, if you use the right techniques.

11

Fitness for great sex

In this chapter you will learn:
- *about food for great sex*
- *how to exercise for great sex*
- *about sex and health.*

You can only respond to sex to the extent that your body allows you to. It doesn't matter how skilful or knowledgeable you or your partner are, if your body doesn't work properly, you won't be able to enjoy the sensations of great sex.

Unfortunately, a lot of people only think about their body's capacity for sex when something starts to go wrong. Then they look for a pill they can take, but you can't put right years of neglect with a pill. That's completely the wrong approach. The right approach is to avoid problems by eating the right food and having proper exercise all your life. Look after your body and your body will look after great sex.

Food and sex

Some doctors believe that about three-quarters of health problems are due to faulty nutrition. Basically, they're saying that you can eat yourself healthy or you can eat yourself ill. And it's certainly true for sex. Sex requires an enormous array of chemicals and a wide-ranging response from the body.

With so many different foods on offer in the supermarket, you'd think you couldn't fail to get every necessary vitamin and mineral in abundance. Not true. So much in the modern diet has had the vital nutrients stripped out. For example, refining whole wheat to white flour loses 86 per cent of the manganese, 85 per cent of the magnesium, 72 per cent of vitamin B6, 67 per cent of the folic acid and 60 per cent of the calcium. It also loses 78 per cent of the zinc which, as you'll see below, is vital to a man's sexual function.

Sexual response may also be impacted by pesticide residues in food, so eat organic whenever you can.

It's a basic requirement that blood should be able to flow freely to the genital region and through all the tiny blood vessels there, for both men and women. Yet a diet high in *saturated* fat (principally animal fat) over the years leads to the deposition of a fatty layer of lipids and low-density lipoprotein (LDL) cholesterol in the blood vessels. Apart from anything else, that's going to make it difficult for erectile tissue to erect.

In fact, circulatory or vascular problems are the most common physical cause of erectile dysfunction. Blood flow into the penis is impaired, leading to a decrease in penile blood pressure. Basically, when you have atherosclerosis (fatty deposits in the arteries) in the pudendal and penile arteries, sufficient blood just can't get through. Women can have a similar problem with the clitoral system.

Part of the answer is to keep the intake of animal fats low. However, cholesterol is also manufactured *in* the body by the liver. Indeed, it's essential to good health (and to having sex), so the situation is complicated. Too much LDL cholesterol is dangerous but, on the other hand, there's a type of cholesterol known as high-density lipoprotein (HDL) that's extremely beneficial. Fortunately, nature has provided foods that can lower LDLs and increase HDLs. Thus, the other part of the answer is to eat these foods:

▶ *Garlic – a couple of raw cloves a day will help keep the blood flowing to your genitals by lowering bad LDL cholesterol. In my focus groups, some men reported that eating garlic when they weren't used to it gave them spontaneous erections. It's the active ingredient allicin that creates the smell, but garlic odour on the breath and on the body diminishes with regular use.*

▶ *Onions – half a raw onion a day will also improve the circulation to the genitals by raising the level of good HDL cholesterol and lowering bad LDL cholesterol. The more pungent the onion, the more powerful the effect. Onions also lower blood sugar thus helping fight diabetes, a cause of impotence.*

▶ *Olive oil – yet another food for improving circulation to the genitals. A smear gives the skin a nice sheen, a dollop lets your bodies slide over one another very enjoyably and, at a pinch, you can use it as a lubricant (not with condoms).*

▶ *Barley and oats – two more powerful foods for raising good HDL cholesterol and lowering bad LDL cholesterol.*

▶ *Beans – these combat haemorrhoids, which are hardly conducive to great sex. Soybeans are rich in natural oestrogen, which makes them important for women going through the menopause and after. (For that reason men may prefer to consume rather less than their partners.)*

▶ *Broccoli, pomegranate and tomatoes – these protect against prostate cancer; broccoli also reduces the incidence of cancer of the cervix in women.*

▶ *Cranberries – a chemical in them somehow envelops the bacteria that cause cystitis (a common urinary infection in women, especially after vigorous sex) and prevents them getting a foothold in the bladder.*

▶ *Seaweed – the Laminaria species in particular protects against breast cancer.*

▶ *Nuts, seeds and dried fruits – important sources of L-arginine, a major constituent of semen and also required for the production of nitric oxide, which causes erection by vasodilation (the widening of blood vessels).*

Remember, the three rules are:

1 *Eat whole and unprocessed foods as much as possible.*
2 *Eat organic whenever possible.*
3 *Avoid saturated fats.*

Insight

Sugar is responsible for a lot of health problems but there is at least one situation in which it can be beneficial. Sex. Guys, something sugary a quarter of an hour beforehand will facilitate an increase in the level of serotonin in your brain, making you feel calmer and reducing any tendency to premature ejaculation. The optimum dose is around 50 g (2 oz) of chocolate.

Insight

The average Western diet is deficient in zinc. Men with inadequate zinc don't produce enough testosterone and can even become impotent. What's the biggest natural source of zinc? Why, oysters, which have long been considered an aphrodisiac.

Moreover, zinc concentration in a normal prostate gland is three to ten times higher than in other tissues. In the cancerous prostate, on the other hand, zinc levels are very low. It seems that malignant prostate cells are unable to accumulate it. There is evidence that a high zinc intake, as it were, forces the malignant cells to take up zinc and, in so doing, to increase apoptosis, which is the process of programmed cell death.

Zinc is vital. Other natural sources include beef liver, wheatgerm, whole grains, brewer's yeast, yeast extracts, nuts and soya, but even if you eat a lot of these you probably still won't be getting enough unless you also eat oysters (85 g (30 z) will give you 63 mg of zinc).

Many people don't eat oysters, so I recommend you take a zinc supplement (and, in the long term, you'll need to balance it with a little extra copper). Around 15 mg of zinc a day and 1 mg of copper is right for most people, but always check with your doctor if you are on any other medication.

Drink and sex

Water is vital to sex as well as to life. The body, after all, is mostly water as are sperm and vaginal secretions. A 2 per cent deficiency of water in the cells is enough to make your brain feel fuzzy. Some experts say our fluid intake should be at least 2.5 litres (4.5 pints) a day, but that's probably excessive, except in hot weather. Tea and coffee count towards the total but alcohol doesn't. The best guide is the colour of your urine. If it's clear to pale straw then it's fine.

As for alcohol, a small quantity may relax you but every mouthful also diminishes sexual response. In the long term, alcohol abuse can lead to erectile dysfunction. Sex is better without it, except for a shared glass of wine afterwards (not before) as explained in Chapter 10.

The anti-sex factory

Just about everybody nowadays realizes that being overweight means an increased risk of heart disease, high blood pressure and diabetes. Rather fewer people realize that these problems and/or their treatment can cause an impairment to sexual capacity. Furthermore, almost nobody knows that a man's paunch is actually an 'anti-sex factory'.

In a man, fat cells around the middle cause excess production of something called 'aromatase enzyme' which converts testosterone to oestrogen. Testosterone is the 'male' sex hormone while oestrogen is the 'female' sex hormone. The result is anything from mild erectile dysfunction to complete impotence. There are two rules:

1 *Keep down the level of saturated fat in your meals – it immediately lowers testosterone for up to four hours.*
2 *Keep your Body Mass Index (BMI) at 24 or lower. Working out your BMI isn't too difficult, but you will need a calculator unless you're very good at maths. It's your weight in*

kilograms divided by your height in metres squared (that's to say, your height in metres multiplied by itself).

Example

You weigh 58 kilos and are 1.6 metres tall. The square of 1.6 (1.6 × 1.6) is 2.56. So your BMI is 58 divided by 2.56 which is 22.6. That's well under 24 and fine. (If you only know your weight in pounds you can convert to kilograms by dividing by 2.2; and to convert inches to metres divide by 39.37.)

This is not the place to go into nutrition in detail. If you are overweight, you should study a good book on the subject such as *Lose Weight, Gain Energy, Get Healthy*. I'll just point out that to lose 450 g (1 lb) in a week you'd need to eat 3,500 calories less during the week, or 500 less per day – the equivalent of a pretty large pudding. If you don't like the idea of cutting out pudding, there's another way. It's called *exercise*.

Exercise and sex

Someone who exercises vigorously can eat about 25 per cent more than someone who spends the day sitting around. However, these first exercises below aren't for losing weight or building muscle; they're simply exercises to put you in touch with your body and to improve your agility for sex. Start with a few repetitions and build up from there.

1 Spread squats. *This is a variation on the old 'touch your toes' exercise. Stand with your feet slightly more than shoulder width apart and, with your legs slightly bent, bend over and place your hands on your feet. Now gradually straighten your legs as much as you can. This is your start position. From this position, with your head hanging, squat down then raise yourself once again into the start position, stretching your legs as much as you can. Exhale as you go down; inhale as you come up.*

2 Butterfly. *Sit on the floor with your thighs open, your knees bent and your feet pressed together by their soles and pulled*

back towards your groin. Put your hands on your feet. Your start position is sitting up with your spine straight and your chest out. Now, bend forward, exhaling, to drop your head as close to your toes as you can manage. Inhale as you return to the start position.

3 Cat-cow. *Get on the floor on your hands and knees. This is the start position. From here raise your head and arch your back so that your stomach curves down towards the floor. Inhale as you do so. Now bend your spine in the opposite direction by rounding your back and dropping your head. Exhale as you do so.*

4 The bow. *Lie on your stomach. Bend your knees and bring your feet as close to your buttocks as you can manage, so that you can reach behind and grab your ankles. Now begin to straighten your legs so that your body is pulled into an arch. This is your start position. Rock backwards, inhaling, then forwards, exhaling. Relax for three minutes.*

5 The locust. *Lie on your stomach. Clench your hands and slide them under your hips either side of your pubic triangle. With your feet together, inhale as you raise your legs behind you, keeping them as straight as possible. Now 'belly breathe' so that your stomach expands as you breathe in and contracts as you breathe out. After 30 seconds, inhale and raise your legs even higher. Slowly return your legs to the floor and relax for three minutes.*

6 The bridge. *Lie on your back with the soles of your feet on the floor, knees bent, and your arms stretched comfortably along the floor past your head, palms upwards. This is your start position. Now inhale as you lift your pelvis and back off the floor and hold for a few seconds. Exhale as you come back down.*

7 Rolling. *Lie on your back and make yourself into a 'ball' by bringing your knees towards your chest and your head towards your knees, locking everything in place with your hands around your lower legs. Now roll backwards and forwards for one minute.*

8 Sex nerves. *Lie on your back, thighs apart, knees bent and the soles of your feet together. Inhale as you stroke your inner*

thighs from your knees up to your groin. Think of sucking up energy into your genitals. Exhale as you return your hands to your knees but without touching yourself.

COUPLES' EXERCISES

Exercising together is a fun and intimate way of improving your co-ordination as a couple. You can make these exercises part of a bigger exercise routine, or incorporate them into your love play.

1 Trees in the wind. *Press against one another, standing up and facing each other. One of you place your hands on your partner's shoulders; the other place your hands around your partner's lower back. Now, sway backwards and forwards, keeping closely together and slowly inhaling and exhaling with the movement.*

2 Squats. *Stand a little apart, facing one another with your feet spread to shoulder width. Grasp your partner's arms just above the wrists, bend your knees and lean back. Now exhale and both slowly squat down. Inhale as you come up.*

3 Back squats. *Standing back to back, interlock your arms at the elbows. Now exhale and slowly squat as far as you can without pushing one another over. Inhale as you come up.*

4 Standing arches. *Standing back to back, interlock your arms at the elbows. With knees bent one of you now leans forward, stretching the other over his or her back. The toes of the partner being stretched should not leave the ground. Hold the position and breathe deeply. Now do it the opposite way.*

5 Leg stretch. *Sit facing one another, legs wide open. The shorter of you places his or her feet against the other's ankles. Now grip each other's wrists. Take turns leaning back and pulling the other forward.*

MORE VIGOROUS EXERCISE

In a Gallup survey, 45 per cent of respondents said their sex lives improved when they began exercising. If that's not a good reason to exercise, I don't know what is.

Exercise strengthens your heart, your respiratory system, your muscles and your bones. You'll have more energy, you'll sleep better, and withstand stress more easily. You'll feel more self-confident, you'll have fewer medical problems, you'll age more slowly and remain active longer, and you'll probably lose weight. On top of all that, you'll boost your levels of endorphins and noradrenaline/norepinephrine, which will make you feel good, plus phenylethylamine (PEA), the same chemical that gives you that 'walking on air' feeling when you fall in love.

What kind of exercise? Well, running is pretty good. Apart from the shorts and the running shoes (and a sports bra for women), it doesn't cost anything and you can do it just about anywhere, either alone or with friends. This is an aerobic activity which means that it reduces the risk of heart disease and some forms of cancer, lowers bad LDL cholesterol in the bloodstream, boosts the immune system, reduces blood pressure, and fights osteoporosis. In terms of losing weight, you'll burn about 100 calories every km (0.6 miles).

If you think running is 'boring', then you could also try aerobic dancing, cycling, football, swimming, squash or tennis... There's plenty to choose from. The important thing is to exercise for at least 20 minutes and to do so a minimum of three times a week. You also need to develop flexibility and improve muscular strength. If you can't match the following, then get exercising straight away:

- ▶ Flexibility. *You should be able to touch your toes sitting on the floor with your legs out straight.*
- ▶ Muscular fitness. *In one minute you should be able to do the following number of push-ups:*
  - ▷ *men in their twenties – around 30*
  - ▷ *men in their thirties – around 25*
  - ▷ *men in their forties – around 20*
  - ▷ *men in their fifties and over – 15.*

  Women are allowed to do push-ups while kneeling, but keeping a flat back and the hips down. The figures for women are:
  - ▷ *in their twenties – around 25*
  - ▷ *in their thirties – around 20*

> ▷ *in their forties – around 15*
> ▷ *in their fifties – around 13*
> ▷ *in their sixties or over – around 8.*
► Aerobic capacity. *Walk 0.8 km (0.5 miles). Men in their twenties and thirties should be able to do it in around six to seven minutes. Men in their forties and fifties should be aiming for seven to eight minutes. Men over 60 should aim for eight to nine minutes. Young women shouldn't be more than a few seconds behind the men but by the time you reach your sixties, ladies, you can allow yourselves an extra minute.*

THE BODY BEAUTIFUL

So far I have talked about fitness, but if you want a beautiful body, a *sculpted* body, the only solution is weight training. The best way to weight train is by joining a gym where there are various machines and proper instruction. If you prefer, machines are available for home use. You can also use free weights (dumb-bells).

► Machines. *You don't have to worry about dropping weights on yourself or anybody else; a well-designed machine puts you in the right position and minimizes the risk of injury.*
► Free weights. *Extremely flexible – you can exercise just about any muscle. They're also more natural and more realistic to everyday life. Free weights are good for balance. They are cheap to buy and use at home, but there is a greater risk of injury or improper technique.*

Guidelines
► *Have proper instruction – you can easily hurt yourself if you don't know the correct way to use the equipment.*

- ▶ Warm up before tackling heavier weights.
- ▶ Do your weight training two to three times a week, with a minimum of one day's rest between sessions – less is not enough, more can be harmful.
- ▶ Heavier weights and fewer repetitions equals visible muscle; lighter weights and more repetitions equals speed and endurance with less visible muscle. Err on the side of lighter weights to avoid injury.
- ▶ A session should be 20–40 minutes long.

KEEPING MOTIVATED

It can be very difficult to keep motivated, no matter how much good you know the exercise is doing you. Once you stop exercising, even if it's just for a couple of weeks, it's harder to get started again. The good news is that results can come very quickly. If you've been fairly sedentary, then you should be able to get into reasonable shape within three months. From zero you could be running a marathon in a year.

Here are some suggestions for keeping the interest going:

- ▶ Don't let the weather put you off – have alternatives for when it's too hot or too cold or too wet for your preferred sport.
- ▶ Exercise with friends, so you can encourage one another.
- ▶ Hang a picture on the wall showing the body you're aiming for.
- ▶ Enjoy your exercise – don't make it a chore.
- ▶ Play music while exercising at home.
- ▶ Set measurable and attainable goals, and celebrate when you reach them.
- ▶ Keep an exercise diary.
- ▶ Make a list of all the exercise benefits you're hoping for, and look at it regularly.

Insight

You can lose weight by eating fewer calories, exercising more or a combination of both. The magic figure to remember is that 3,500 calories is equivalent to 450 g (1 lb) of body weight. Walk 45 minutes a day and at the end of a year you'll have lost 11 kg (24 lb). To achieve the same through diet, you'll have to eat 230 fewer calories a day (equivalent to an average pudding).

EXERCISING THE PC MUSCLE

I've already talked about the importance of exercising the group of muscles popularly known as the 'PC muscle' (Chapters 2 and 3). In men, this muscle assists in and gives force to orgasm and ejaculation, and can be used consciously to flex the penis inside the vagina. In women, the PC muscle assists orgasm, contributes to a tight vagina, and can be used to squeeze and massage the penis inside the vagina (a technique known as *kabazzah*).

It's very easy for both men and women to exercise their PC muscles. It is the muscle you would use to stop the flow of urine when urinating. You can flex it quite invisibly, which means that you can exercise it at any time. A basic exercise is to contract the muscle, hold for one to two seconds, then release. Repeat ten times several times a day.

In women, weakness of the PC muscle leads, in extreme cases, to leakage of urine or incontinence. The female anatomy gives women an advantage over men when exercising the PC muscle because it's very easy for them to introduce a resistance for exercise. One of the oldest methods used is the stone egg, which dates back thousands of years. Jade is particularly attractive but you can also buy eggs in stainless steel and other materials.

The idea is to pop a lubricated egg into the vagina and then use the vaginal muscles to move it up and down. Squeezing the perineum and vagina moves the egg up, while bearing down (as for a bowel movement) sends it down and out.

Another style involves squeezing against a moveable resistance. An easy way of providing such a resistance is to insert two lubricated fingers into your vagina, open them (as if making a V-sign) and then try to force them closed, using your vagina (and, therefore, your PC muscle). Begin with, say, ten contractions three times a day and work up to 50 contractions three times a day.

A problem with all these kinds of exercises is that it's difficult to know how you're doing. Which, in turn, means it's hard to keep motivated. Dr Arnold Kegel not only devised exercises as a non-surgical method of tackling urinary stress incontinence, but actually invented an apparatus back in 1947 (the Kegel Perineometer) which provided a resistance together with a dial to give biofeedback. Dr Kegel is now dead and his machine is no longer available, but modern 'Kegel' devices are being manufactured. In essence, they're the plastic equivalent of two fingers, hinged together and with a series of springs between. Look for a model capable of providing a dozen different levels of resistance and made with high-quality materials (stainless steel for the springs).

For men, there are prostate massagers that also help to tone the PC muscle. If you're doing exercises without the help of any apparatus, you'll need to follow a fairly involved programme. The exercises below get harder as they go on.

▶ *Contract and release your PC muscle as many times as possible in ten seconds. Repeat three times with breaks of ten seconds in between. As you get better, increase the number of contractions per session and the number of sessions per day.*
▶ *Slowly contract and then hold your PC muscle for five seconds. Repeat ten times initially, building up to 50 times a day.*
▶ *After warming up with short contractions, slowly squeeze and hold your PC muscle as tightly as possible for 30 seconds. Rest and repeat five times. Over a few weeks aim to build up the period for which you can hold your PC muscle to as much as two minutes.*
▶ *Instead of steadily increasing and releasing the contraction, do it in five steps, holding for five seconds at each intermediate stage and for 30 seconds at maximum contraction. This will help improve control.*

Massage for sexual health

In Chapter 4 we took a look at massage as a prelude to sex.
Here, we're more concerned with sexual health.

Everybody knows about the circulation of the blood. Less well-
known is the circulation of lymphatic fluid that fights disease,
eliminates toxins and shifts fat. The lymphatic system has no
pump; it relies entirely on activity of the muscles. In other words,
if you're not getting much exercise, your lymphatic system may get
clogged up.

This is where a therapeutic massage can help. Warm up with
the massage techniques described in Chapter 4 (page 78), giving
plenty of *effleurage*. Then introduce the additional technique of
intermittent pressure. Lymph fluid is what's known as 'thixotropic'.
That's to say that it can exist in either a liquid or a gel form. When
you press hard it turns to gel and doesn't move easily. So, you have
to press gently with your fingers and palms, both downwards and
in the direction the lymph needs to travel from the hands towards
the shoulders and from the feet towards the groin. Press several
times before moving on.

When it comes to sex, the groin is the most important area. There
are several lymph nodes situated in the crease between the thigh
and the abdomen. In a healthy person, one or more can just be

felt, like little peas below the surface. If they're enlarged or painful then a blockage is indicated. Gently work your way along from the genitals up the crease towards the hip bone. (This is something you can do for yourself if your partner isn't available.) Then, from the middle of the crease work your way diagonally up towards the navel and then straight up to the breast bone.

If you're not going to have sex, there's an excellent way of ending the massage that involves building tension throughout the body then abruptly releasing it. At an agreed moment, the person doing the massaging ceases all touching, and their partner takes several deep breaths then holds one breath and clenches every possible muscle for ten seconds. It helps to raise the legs, arms and torso for maximum tension. The partner then completely relaxes and breathes normally. The effect is enhanced if he or she wears an eye mask and if there's some soft music playing.

Insight

The penis can be included in a massage. Use a little evening primrose oil to improve the elasticity of the skin, gently stroking it in from the base towards the tip. For more on penis massage see Chapter 14.

Smoking and sex

If you smoke, the quickest thing you can do to improve your sex life is give up right now. An Australian study has shown that smoking up to 20 cigarettes a day increases the likelihood of impotence by 24 per cent compared with non-smokers. Men who smoke more than 20 a day have a 40 per cent higher risk of impotence than non-smokers. A different study has put the figure at 50 per cent.

The British Medical Association has estimated that up to 120,000 men in their thirties and forties in the UK are impotent as a direct result of smoking. Smoking impairs the erection process. It also impairs the valve mechanism that traps blood in the penis, reduces the volume of ejaculate (and therefore the satisfaction), lowers the sperm count, and impairs the sperm.

As if you needed any more encouragement to give up, smokers lose more teeth than non-smokers. In fact, data from the Centers for Disease Control and Prevention in the USA showed that over 40 per cent of smokers were toothless by the age of 65, compared with around 20 per cent of non-smokers. Basically, smoking causes gums to recede, increases plaque, causes pockets between teeth and gums and destroys the bone and tissue that support the teeth. Not much fun when it comes to kissing.

10 THINGS TO REMEMBER

1 *Excellent foods for a healthy sex life include garlic, onions, olive oil, beans, barley, oats, broccoli, pomegranate, tomatoes, cranberries, seaweed, nuts, seeds and dried fruits.*

2 *In general, favour whole, unprocessed foods to ensure a good supply of vitamins and minerals.*

3 *Foods to avoid include those high in saturated fats (which can lower testosterone for four hours and can cause long-term damage to blood circulation in the genitals) and those with high pesticide residues (which can interfere with sexual response).*

4 *A zinc supplement is advisable for men's sexual health.*

5 *A man's paunch is an 'anti-sex factory', converting testosterone to oestrogen.*

6 *For great sex, keep your BMI at 24 or less.*

7 *Water is essential to great sex but alcohol and smoking equal bad sex.*

8 *Gentle stretches prepare the body for sex right now; regular, vigorous exercise will keep you prepared for sex always.*

9 *For a beautiful body, try weight lifting; for a beautiful vagina/penis work that PC muscle.*

10 *Massage can improve health and sexual response.*

HOW GREAT IS SEX NOW?

▶ *Have you switched to the 'great sex' way of eating?*   Yes/No

▶ *If you have a BMI above 24, have you begun a*
  programme to reduce it?   Yes/No

▶ *Are you doing those 'sexercises'?*   Yes/No

▶ *Are you generating PEA and the other feel-good*
  chemicals with a regular exercise regime?   Yes/No

▶ *Are you giving weight lifting a go?*   Yes/No

▶ *Are you exercising your PC muscle every day (right*
  now, for example)?   Yes/No

▶ *Are you a non-smoker?*   Yes/No

▶ *Do you drink only in moderation (or less)?*   Yes/No

If you answered 'no' to more than three questions, re-read the
relevant parts of the chapter and make an effort to put the
suggestions into effect. Talking about sensible eating and exercise
can seem rather boring compared with sex, but you can't divorce
your sexual ability from your general health and fitness. And
looking at it from the opposite perspective, better sex is a great
incentive to start on that exercise programme. Try to engage your
partner in everything as well – it's easier when you're both pulling
together. Fix your mind on the benefits – they'll come very quickly
in terms of sexual performance.

12

....

Great sex during and after pregnancy

In this chapter you will learn:
- *when it's safe to have sex*
- *the techniques and benefits of sex during pregnancy*
- *how to restore your body after the birth.*

Creating a child is an incredibly special thing, which most people only do twice in a lifetime. It's a process so amazing that modern science can't fully explain it, miraculous if not actually a miracle. But pregnancy can be a demanding time for both of you, so when the going gets tough reflect upon the marvel that it is. Continuing to have a great sex life can help quite a lot.

Sex during pregnancy

Pregnancy isn't a time for giving up sex. On the contrary, it's when you need plenty of oxytocin, the hormone that binds you together. And, as you've seen, oxytocin is released during sex. There are also other important reasons to continue your sex life:

▶ *Sex can help release the physical tensions that pregnancy creates.*
▶ *Sex can help discharge any feelings of resentment between you.*

- *Sex can help reassure a man that he's not become less important.*
- *Sex can help reassure a woman that she's still desirable.*
- *Sex can be comforting.*
- *Sex is great.*

However, although you can and should continue your sex life together, you're going to have to prepare for the idea that it's going to be very *different*.

In terms of sex, during the pregnancy and after can be divided into four phases:

1 *First three months – occasional intercourse, oral sex, mutual masturbation.*
2 *The next four months – great sex; multiple orgasms for women.*
3 *The final two months plus the six weeks following the birth – for her, some gentle sex prior to the birth but afterwards none until approved by a health professional; for him, fellatio, solo masturbation, experimentation with multiple orgasms.*
4 *The next six months – gradual return to normal libido and response.*

Approach each phase in a positive way. Don't look upon pregnancy as lost time for sex; look upon it as a great time for experimentation, for trying new ways of giving one another physical pleasure and comfort. Of course, pregnancy is also a time for lots of kissing and cuddling and reassurance. Have a look again at some of the ideas in Chapter 4.

IS IT SAFE?

Your first concern will probably be the safety of the baby. Is it really appropriate to be thrusting away right under the baby's nose, as it were? In fact, it's not only okay, it's recommended. Remember that intercourse takes place in the vagina, while the baby is snugly ensconced in the uterus, protected by the cervix and a little bag of amniotic fluid. Foetuses have been observed while women are having orgasms and absolutely no signs of distress have been noted.

Yet, there are certain things that are dangerous during pregnancy:

► *Never blow air into the vagina of a pregnant woman because it can kill both her and the baby within minutes. It happens because air blown into the vagina can pass beneath the foetal membranes and into the circulation of what are known as the 'subplacental sinuses' resulting in air embolism (air bubbles in the blood that stop the circulation). In fact, never blow air into any woman. It's pointless (and can you be certain she's not pregnant?). Some doctors are so worried by the possibility of embolism they advise against oral sex entirely during pregnancy.*

► *As a pregnant woman, you should never have sex unless you're positive that your partner is free of any sexually transmitted disease (STD). Apart from the risk to you, STDs can be extremely dangerous to your developing baby.*

FIRST THREE MONTHS

If it's a woman's first pregnancy, she probably won't be very interested in sex during this time. She'll quite likely be worried that sex may damage the baby (it won't), and she will feel sick and tired. Most women find that subsequent pregnancies don't affect their sex drive and response so much, unless they have morning sickness.

Nevertheless, even a woman pregnant for the first time will feel like intercourse occasionally. Her breasts will enlarge considerably during the first three months, which will excite her partner quite a lot, and she may feel somewhat proud of them and want to show them off. Take care as they will be rather tender. During sex the breasts will enlarge even further.

When a woman is interested in sex but doesn't feel like intercourse, try being a human armchair (see Chapter 4) in which she can masturbate or you can stimulate her clitoris. You can both enjoy oral sex.

THE NEXT FOUR MONTHS

From about the end of the third month of the pregnancy, things are usually rather different. Women tend to want sex. If this is the case with you, you'll quite likely spend a lot of time daydreaming about great sex. Enjoy your fantasies. You may even find that real sex is better than ever before. Two of six women being studied by William Masters and Virginia Johnson actually *became* multi-orgasmic during this period. It probably has a lot to do with the vasocongestion that naturally builds up: this is the same kind of engorgement of the blood vessels that occurs during sex anyway and it means that a woman already has a head start. There's also naturally more lubrication. At this stage orgasms will be as powerful as before and feel good, but they might bring on backache and cramp.

THE FINAL TWO MONTHS PLUS THE SIX WEEKS FOLLOWING THE BIRTH

As a woman approaches seven months in her pregnancy, she'll probably find that her orgasms seem less powerful and no longer relieve her tension as they did. Intercourse in just about any position is increasingly uncomfortable. Her abdomen will be hugely distended and, although her breasts will be about one-third bigger, she won't feel much like having them played with. Basically, she just won't feel very sexy. But, if occasionally she does, intercourse is still possible.

It's true that at one time pregnant women were told as a matter of routine to avoid sex during the last six weeks. Nowadays, the professional view is that sex is safe during all stages of a 'normal' pregnancy, unless there are particular problems, including:

▶ *a history of miscarriage or a medical condition with an increased risk of miscarriage, because orgasm and prostaglandins in the semen could trigger contractions (However, at least one study found that orgasms were associated with lower rates of premature birth.)*

▸ *a history of premature delivery or signs that delivery might be premature*
▸ *any unexplained vaginal discharge, bleeding or pain*
▸ *loss of amniotic fluid (the fluid that surrounds the baby)*
▸ *placenta previa (a condition in which the placenta covers the cervix)*
▸ *weak cervix*
▸ *twins (or more).*

The question of safety following the birth is very different. The vagina will have had a pretty traumatic time. It may actually get torn and, in any event, there will be bleeding for two to four weeks. Consequently, *until a doctor has given the all clear* (which will probably be at the time of the woman's full medical check-up when the baby is around six weeks old), you should follow these guidelines:

▸ No *intercourse.*
▸ No *other kind of penetrative sex (e.g. using fingers).*
▸ No *cunnilingus (because it may cause infection).*
▸ No *blowing into the vagina (because it can still cause an air embolism – and don't do it at any other time, either).*

Guys, don't look upon this whole period without intercourse (which often lasts three months) as a burden. Look upon it as a great time to experiment with your own body. If you're not yet multi-orgasmic then read Chapter 8 again and spend this period practising. It's an ideal time; since your partner can't have intercourse there's no problem if you ejaculate by mistake while experimenting.

A great idea, when your partner feels like it, is to masturbate side by side or sitting at opposite ends of the bed, watching one another. The reason for this is that oxytocin can't work its magic of binding you together if you masturbate separately. Women produce oxytocin as soon as stimulation begins, but men produce it immediately before ejaculation. By learning how to have multiple orgasms during masturbation with your partner and approaching ejaculation several times, a man can increase the amount of oxytocin without experiencing the sexual hangover later.

If your partner is willing, this is also a great opportunity to experiment with fellatio to orgasm/ejaculation.

THE NEXT SIX MONTHS

Some men are so traumatized by seeing their partners suffer during childbirth that they're actually put off sex for a while. At the same time, some women, who may not have had sex for several months, find it difficult to get back into it. This is all the more so if there's fear about another pregnancy. These negative feelings usually pass, but if they don't then speak to a health professional.

When, with the doctor's approval, you do resume intercourse, you'll notice that some things are different for a while. A woman won't lubricate as quickly (so have a lubricant handy), and it'll take longer for vasocongestion to build up. Orgasms will be shorter and less intense. Milk may spurt from the breasts, and they won't enlarge as they used to.

Incidentally, breastfeeding is another way of releasing oxytocin, which helps bind mother and baby together. In fact, many women find that breastfeeding is itself sexually exciting and occasionally even leads to orgasm. If this is the case, don't feel guilty about it because it's perfectly normal. Breastfeeding also increases a woman's prolactin level, which can decrease sexual desire. On the other hand, some studies have found that women who breastfeed recover their libidos the quickest – so the evidence isn't clear on this.

Guys, ensure you're part of this 'love-in' as well. When you're not having much sex (your partner is still going to be exhausted a lot of the time), continue masturbating together with her and having multiple orgasms. Make sure that you, too, bond with the baby by taking part in everything and having plenty of physical contact.

By the end of this six months, a woman's libido and response should be back to normal. And if the man has been practising as recommended, then their sex life together will be better than ever.

Techniques during pregnancy

As I've stressed all through the book, there are plenty of sexual things that you can do other than have intercourse. These other techniques can become more important during pregnancy when a woman may just feel too exhausted or uncomfortable. Have a look back at Chapter 5. This is the time for lots of oral stimulation (but note the warning about blowing air into a vagina above), mutual masturbation and side-by-side masturbation.

As the pregnancy develops, so some of the positions that were easy before become uncomfortable and eventually impossible. Choose positions that don't put weight on the woman, that don't require the woman to support her own weight entirely and that either favour shallow penetration or, at least, allow the woman to control the depth of penetration.

My focus groups have rated the following positions on a scale of one to 100, and they're listed here in order of popularity. I've left a space for you to add your own score.

THE IMPROVED MISSIONARY POSITION

This was the most popular position among non-pregnant women in my focus groups and also rated the best by those in the earlier stages of pregnancy. The important thing is for the woman to have sufficient pillows under her buttocks so that the man can either kneel or squat. This way, there's no pressure on her. Alternatively, the woman can lie on the bed with her vulva at the edge and her feet on the floor; the man can stand, kneel or squat, depending on the height of the bed.

Focus group score: 90   Your score: ....

THE T VARIANT

This is a variation on the T position in Chapter 6 (page 137). The woman lies on her back with her knees bent and her feet on the bed. The man lies on his side and *sideways* to her, with his hips by her feet. Raising her legs, he now drapes them over himself as he eases himself forward. This is a gentle position in which the woman has no weight on her at all and in which the depth of penetration is easily controlled.

Focus group score: 80   Your score: ....

THE SITTING EMBRACE, VARIATION 2

This position, fully described in Chapter 6 (page 124), is particularly tender at this time. The man sits on the bed and the woman sits on his lap with her legs around him. You can look into one another's eyes and think about the wonderful things that are going on in your lives together. Movement is difficult, especially when the pregnancy is advanced, but this is an excellent posture for prolonged lovemaking.

Focus group score: 80   Your score: ....

SPOONS

The woman simply lies on her side with her thighs approximately at right angles to her body and her knees bent. The man enters her from behind. To stop air being pumped into the vagina, penetration should be shallow and thrusting gentle. The man should withdraw from time to time so that any trapped air can escape. As with the Improved missionary, the woman can, as a variation, lie with her buttocks at the edge of the bed and the man can stand, kneel or squat, depending on the height of the bed.

Focus group score: 80   Your score: ....

PASSERS BY

The woman lies on her side, roughly in a banana shape. The man then enters from behind but, as it were, upside down with *his face close to her feet*. This is a comfortable position for both which makes it easy for the man to stimulate the woman's G-spot while she can stimulate her own clitoris.

Focus group score: 75   Your score: ....

THE AMAZON

The man lies on his side. The woman raises his upper leg and kneels astride his lower thigh, facing him. Like this she can control the depth of penetration and rub her clitoris against him.

Focus group score: 75   Your score: ....

THE TRAP DOOR

This is the opposite of the Amazon. The woman lies on her side. The man then raises her upper leg and kneels astride her lower thigh, facing her.

Focus group score: 70   Your score: ....

Your relationship

Hopefully, before the pregnancy you had a happy relationship and were both equally committed to having a baby. However, even the strongest relationships come under pressure during pregnancy and its aftermath.

It's only common sense that when there's a baby around you'll have less time for one another. And, even in the most egalitarian of households, it's usually the woman who looks after the baby the most. This can mean that the woman feels resentful about having to do so much of the work while the man gets resentful about getting less attention.

Men don't get pregnant, they don't endure childbirth, and they rarely share the burden of a baby equally with their partners. So, incredible as it may seem, it may be the case that they really don't understand what it's like for a woman.

It's important for a man to be involved in all the medical discussions for the pregnancy and birth right from the very beginning. A man may not believe it when his partner tells him that, for example, even cunnilingus is forbidden. This is where a few words from the doctor can be helpful for both of you.

A man can feel jealous of the baby, particularly so if it's a boy. Suddenly, there's a new man in his partner's life and he may find that hard. Of course, the mother's relationship with the baby is something very different, but some men may fail to understand the distinction.

As a man, the best thing you can do to start enjoying great sex again is to be understanding and to give your partner as much physical and moral support as possible. For both your sakes, you need to have time together and to relate to one another as you did before. This doesn't mean withdrawing from the turmoil at home but throwing yourself into it. Enlist as much help as you can from other members of the family as well. Make sure your partner gets enough sleep and eats properly. If she doesn't have time for these essentials, she's more likely to suffer some form of post-natal depression. In fact, half to two-thirds of new mothers suffer the 'baby blues', while between 10 and 15 per cent suffer more serious post-natal depression. So, look after her.

Permanent changes

Once a woman has given birth, there may be some small but permanent changes to her body. These are perfectly normal, and they won't interfere with sexual enjoyment. There will be extra enlargement of the outer labia during sexual excitement, and this may even heighten arousal for both of you. The uterus, too, will enlarge more than it did, but that's invisible.

However, a woman who's breast-fed one baby won't experience as much enlargement during sexual excitement as she used to. If she's breast-fed two or more she may not experience any enlargement at all. The explanation seems to be that suckling increases the ability of the breasts to carry blood away so that vasocongestion no longer occurs.

The vagina, having expanded to allow a baby to pass, won't immediately feel as tight as it used to. The solution is to begin PC exercises, as described in Chapter 11, as soon as a health professional says it's safe to do so. In fact, there's no reason why a woman can't have an even stronger PC muscle than before she was pregnant.

10 THINGS TO REMEMBER

1 *Sex during pregnancy helps to bind partners together.*

2 *Intercourse is safe at all stages of a normal pregnancy, but a doctor may tell you to stop if there are complications.*

3 *During the first three months of pregnancy, 'first-timers' generally don't feel much like sex, but women who've been pregnant before usually maintain their libidos.*

4 *During the following four months, most pregnant women feel more like sex than ever before due to the permanent vasocongestion of the pelvic area.*

5 *The two months prior to the birth and the six weeks after (when intercourse isn't possible) is a great time for men to learn to become multi-orgasmic.*

6 *Men should be involved in the medical discussions so they can hear the advice for themselves.*

7 *Men who experience multiple orgasms while masturbating with their partners will feel a powerful bond from the hormone oxytocin.*

8 *There are special positions you can use for intercourse during pregnancy.*

9 *Don't neglect your relationship once a baby has come along.*

10 *The tightness of the vagina can be restored by PC muscle exercises.*

HOW GREAT IS SEX NOW?

▶ *Are you continuing to have a sex life with your*
  partner during pregnancy?   Yes/No

▶ *Are you enjoying plenty of intercourse during months*
  four to six?   Yes/No

▶ *Have you been experimenting with side-by-side*
  masturbation when intercourse isn't possible?   Yes/No

▶ *Were you able to get back to a normal sex life*
  once the doctor had given the all-clear approximately
  six weeks after the birth?   Yes/No

▶ *Men: have you been using your 'time off' to perfect*
  your technique for multiple orgasms?   Yes/No

▶ *Men: have you been doing your fair share of the work*
  of looking after the baby and running the house?   Yes/No

▶ *Women: once the health professional said it was*
  safe to do so, did you begin a programme of PC
  muscle exercises?   Yes/No

If you answered 'no' to more than three questions, re-read the
relevant parts of the chapter and make an effort to put the
suggestions into effect. Pregnancy can be a wonderful shared
experience for a couple if you do it right.

13

....

Great sex ever after

In this chapter you will learn:
- *how a woman's body changes with age*
- *how a man's body changes with age*
- *how you can continue to enjoy sex at any age.*

Wow! It just keeps on getting better and better. That's the message from most men and women who are over 50. In plenty of cases, *well* over 50.

You see, sex is a little like the economy. If you expect it to go downhill, it will. But if you keep optimistic, it improves. The first thing to get out of your mind is any notion that your sex life is in decline. As I shall prove to you in this chapter, the opposite is the case; your sex life is on the up. Just look at all the advantages of being older:

▶ *more time for sex*
▶ *more knowledge about sex*
▶ *more skill in sex*
▶ *more experimentation in sex*
▶ *more knowledge of your own body*
▶ *more knowledge of your partner's body (assuming you've been together a while)*
▶ *more multi-orgasmic*
▶ *more control over ejaculation*
▶ *less guilt about sex*

- *less inhibition about sex*
- *no fear of pregnancy*
- *no menstruation*
- *no worries about the side effects of contraceptives*
- *no premature ejaculation.*

Women

Most women's sexual pleasure increases with age. Why should this be? One theory is that while women's oestrogen levels fall at menopause, their testosterone levels don't fall so much (women have testosterone too). Just as with men, testosterone plays a role in a woman's sex drive, and when it isn't 'counterbalanced' by so much oestrogen, the libido goes up. In addition, 30 or more years of sexual activity will have increased the system of veins in the genitals, leading to easier orgasms. An older woman is also more skilful and has thrown her inhibitions out of the bedroom window.

Menopause removes the fear of pregnancy and eliminates the need for contraception. If male condoms have been the choice of contraceptive for the last fertile years, then a man is going to notice a substantial increase in stimulation and a woman is going to notice a warmer feeling, increased sensitivity, a contribution to lubrication from him and no more of that funny squeaky sound. Nor is there any longer the need for him to withdraw immediately after ejaculation (in case the condom slips off), so the woman can enjoy the feeling of fullness and contact for longer.

If you're a woman over 50, here are the 'rules' for continuing to enjoy great sex:

- *vibrators*
- *lubrication*
- *frequency*
- *understanding men over 50 (see 'Men' below).*

VIBRATORS

I recommend vibrators to couples of all ages, but at 50 and over a vibrator or two (or three) are vital pieces of equipment. Even though you may orgasm more easily than you did when you were young, a vibrator is still useful to 'wake up' parts of your anatomy that have started to take life easy.

If you already use a vibrator and don't seem to get the stimulation you used to, then switch to a more powerful design. Rigid mains powered models are the best. Some of them can be used all over your body, which is very nice. Be sure to play your vibrator on your clitoris a few minutes before intercourse because that will help with lubrication (see below).

Insight

There are supplements that can help you maintain your sexual and physical form. To slow down age-related muscle loss, try introducing amino acid supplementation to your exercise programme. And to keep the blood flowing in those erectile tissues Vitamin E, Ginkgo biloba and fresh garlic have been shown to be effective.

LUBRICATION

All through this book, I have stressed lubrication for everyone. At 60, you'll be slower to lubricate (one to three minutes on average compared to 10–30 seconds when you were 20), and the quantity will be less. What's more, as you get older so the walls of the vagina become thinner and, as a result, the urethra (which runs along the wall of the vagina) gets irritated when you have sex. If you feel a burning sensation for a day or two after sex when urinating, this (rather than cystitis) could be the reason. This is why extra lubrication is so important because it insulates your urethra.

If you've been relying on saliva as a lubricant, now is the time to treat yourself to the best lubricant for you (and have fun trying them out).

Interestingly, in a William Masters and Virginia Johnson study, two women aged between 61 and 70 and one of 73 all had the lubrication speed of young women. These were the only women to have continued sex at a level of once or twice a week, which brings us to the question of frequency.

FREQUENCY

It is not only faster lubrication that goes with more frequent sex; just about everything is better. Studies have compared older women who had sex at least once a week with older women who had sex only occasionally. The women who had regular sex were still able to enjoy four to seven contractions of the vagina at orgasm compared with three to five for the other women. They showed much higher levels of myotonia (the muscular tension that builds up and is released in orgasm), and were more likely to experience contraction of the rectal sphincter, which is rare after 50. Contractions of the uterus were also more likely. The opening of the outer labia, vasocongestion of the inner labia, sexual flush, breast enlargement, nipple erection and, above all, enlargement of the clitoris were all more apparent in women who had regular sex lives.

I'm not suggesting you have sex once a week. I'm still suggesting you have sex of some kind *every day*. I've already said that daily sex should be the target for couples, and just because you're over 50 there's no reason to cut back. On the contrary, it's even more important to have frequent sex to help prevent ageing. Sex is a form of natural 'hormone replacement therapy'. (However, if you think you do need hormone replacement therapy see Chapter 14.) Of course, in order to achieve that, your partner also has to be capable of sex every day. Don't worry, he almost certainly is, but you have to understand how men over 50 function. That's what we're going to look at next.

Insight
If you're retired, there's no need to squash sex into bedtime as many younger couples have to. Choose a time when you're feeling at your most vigorous. Perhaps mid-morning or, more likely, mid-afternoon. Be decadent.

Men

It was Mark Twain who wrote that the sexual performance of a man over 50 'is of poor quality, the intervals between are wide, and its satisfactions of no great value to either party'. Well, that's all he knew. To be fair to the famous author, he was writing 100 years ago when people aged faster, only a very few had access to the secrets of great sex, and things like PC strengthening exercises were unheard of.

Nowadays, men talking about their sex lives from 50 onwards use the word 'different' a great deal but, unlike Mark Twain, they don't find it lacks satisfaction. On the contrary, they say that quality is up but frequency is down. Well, that's half good. In fact, there are techniques for maintaining not just quality but frequency as well, and we'll come to those in a moment. First of all, if you're a man over 50, here are the 'rules' for continuing to enjoy great sex:

- ▶ *erotica and solo masturbation*
- ▶ *lubrication*
- ▶ *masturbation with your partner*
- ▶ *frequency*
- ▶ *Tao.*

EROTICA AND SOLO MASTURBATION

Malcolm Muggeridge wrote that pornography's aim of exciting sexual desire was 'unnecessary in the case of the young, inconvenient in the case of the middle aged, and unseemly in the old'. Wittily expressed but wrong on every count.

As you get older your testosterone level does down and, as you've seen, your oestrogen level goes up. In Chapter 11 we learned one way of keeping testosterone high by getting rid of that paunch. Another technique is to use erotica regularly. It'll increase your testosterone (and sex drive) and, if you masturbate at the same time but not to ejaculation, you'll give it a further boost.

Older men sometimes avoid sex because they're not confident they can get an erection and ejaculate. Masturbating just sufficiently to have an erection is a check on your 'status'.

Insight

I'll have more to say about food supplements in the next chapter on sexual problems but, once past 50, there are particular things you should be doing to make sure you never have a problem. A zinc supplement is essential (as described in Chapter 11) and it's also a good idea to take saw palmetto, which can boost free testosterone and inhibit prostate enlargement. Vitamin E, Ginkgo biloba and fresh garlic will all help keep the blood flowing to those erectile tissues. To help prevent the loss of muscle as the years go by, take amino acids in conjunction with exercise.

LUBRICATION

Yet again I stress the importance of extra lubrication. It will enhance both masturbation and intercourse.

MASTURBATION WITH YOUR PARTNER

Masturbation together with your partner is something else I have recommended in this book, and for a man past 50 it assumes a vital importance. It's essential that you feel free, when necessary, to masturbate during lovemaking if you're having difficulty getting or maintaining a stiff erection. This is just a fact of life. The things that excited you so powerfully when you were 18 just can't be expected to have the same impact 40 years later when you've seen and experienced them thousands of times. Hopefully, your partner will be ready with oral sex and her fingers but, sometimes, only you can give the necessary stimulation.

Insight

Alcohol has a much worse effect on your sex life when you're older. It will decrease your erections considerably and reduce sensation. So, don't drink when you're going to have sex.

FREQUENCY

If your partner has been reading this book, she's going to want sex every day and you have got to provide it. How?

Age, inevitably, takes its toll on a man's sexual performance. Ejaculation at 50 or so is normally only half the distance that it was when younger and, if erection has been prolonged, the semen only seeps out. Contractions of the rectal sphincter seldom occur. The scrotum becomes less sensitive and experiences less vasocongestion. Moreover, after ejaculation the penis goes down very quickly so there's none of that lying together afterwards, your penis still inside her. Worst of all, the refractory period, during which it isn't possible to have sex, gets longer and longer. You can look upon all this as a negative, if you choose. Or you can look upon it as an opportunity to explore a different style of sex.

One possible solution is to make intercourse as short and sharp as possible. By going for a quickie, your sexual apparatus won't get fatigued. Why not, when you feel like it? However, there is another way, and in my opinion a better way, which is the complete opposite – Tao.

TAO

In many cultures, ejaculation wasn't seen as the high point of sex. It was seen as a failure, a mistake, an error. It meant the pleasures of lovemaking were abruptly ended. It meant, perhaps, giving up an hour of delight in return for sensations that, however pleasurable, lasted only a few seconds.

Possibly nowhere was this philosophy more developed than in the Chinese spiritual tradition of the Tao. The Taoists believed that men should preserve their 'ching', because when a man ejaculated he lost not just semen but his entire vitality, his physical, mental and spiritual energy. As a young man you'd almost certainly have scorned such a notion, but after 50, it may be something you can relate to. You've almost certainly noticed that you can't ejaculate as often as you used to, and when you do ejaculate you probably feel a little 'flat' for a day or so afterwards. You possibly even avoid sex sometimes so that you don't get that feeling of lost vigour.

It would seem that the ability to ejaculate when you're older is related to your ability when you're younger. Shere Hite took data from a man who was still ejaculating five or six times a week at age 64, but that was compared with some 40 ejaculations a week at age 16. The man was something of an exception, of course, but nevertheless the drop of 85 per cent in sexual performance probably holds good for most men. In other words, if you used to ejaculate once a day in your teens, you'll probably be ejaculating once a week by the time you retire.

Sun S'sû-Mo, a Taoist physician born in 581 CE set down the wisdom of the Taoist tradition when he recommended the following frequencies for ejaculation:

▶ *Age 20 – once every four days.*
▶ *Age 30 – once every eight days.*
▶ *Age 40 – once every ten days.*
▶ *Age 50 – once every 20 days.*
▶ *Age 60 – once every 30 days.*

In Taoist thought, the seasons also played a role in ejaculation frequency. Basically, a man could have the most ejaculations in the spring, rather fewer in the summer and none at all in winter.

There are two ways of following the Tao in sex:

1 *Intercourse with orgasm but without ejaculation (multiple orgasms).*
2 *Intercourse without either orgasm or ejaculation.*

I've already written about multiple orgasms in Chapter 8.
If you haven't read it, read it now. Here I'm going to deal with intercourse without either ejaculation or orgasm.

Why on earth, you may ask, would anyone wish to? Well, although older men are usually much better at multiple orgasms than younger men, there can come a time when control mysteriously starts to slip away again. This paradox comes about because of a loss of sensation of the point of no return (PNR). Young men have up to three seconds after the PNR to alert a partner and help her orgasm. In an older man, the time interval between recognizing the PNR and ejaculation shortens to almost nothing. The two-stage ejaculatory pattern of youth becomes one stage.

When and if that happens, it can become easier to have sex without either ejaculation or orgasm. Of course, such lovemaking still requires good control, but it isn't necessary to get infinitely close to the PNR. Call it a fallback plan if you have trouble mastering the technique for multiple orgasms. You won't get the intense sensations that go with multiple orgasms, but you will enjoy all the highly pleasurable experiences that precede that stage and, what's more, for almost *as long as you like*.

> What counts is not arriving, but the journey, and the longer the journey, the better.

If you're not convinced this is going to be enjoyable just ask yourself this: 'What are the things that I enjoy about sex?' Let me make some suggestions. Undressing your partner. Inhaling the perfume of her skin. The physical comfort of your naked bodies hugging. Exciting your partner. Feeling her body tremble in your arms as she has her first orgasm. Feeling your own excitement rise. Giving yourself up to the rapture as the dopamine hits your brain. I could go on, but my point is this: when you feel you can enjoy multiple orgasms, then enjoy multiple orgasms. When you feel you can ejaculate, ejaculate if you wish. But when you have the feeling that you won't be able to do either, why not still enjoy all the other marvellous things about lovemaking? You're not losing anything. You're gaining extra lovemaking sessions.

Some claim that you can have intercourse several times a day by following the Tao. That's not actually true for an older man.

In reality, even though you don't ejaculate, you'll still lose a little fluid. And even if you don't orgasm, various mechanisms in the brain and elsewhere will get fatigued. Yet it is true that you can probably have sex every day, assuming your partner wants to. You won't have any fears over performance and, as a result of that, your performance will probably improve. But how will she feel about the Tao?

Faking it
We hear a lot about women faking orgasm, but as men get older they can start faking too. They find they can't ejaculate so, in order to please their partners, they pretend to. For obvious reasons it's not easy to get away with, but it is an approximation of the way of the Tao. Much better, though, is for you both to discuss the effects of ageing and agree that the Tao is a more appropriate style of lovemaking. Be completely frank and open because, only in that way, can you both fully enjoy yourselves.

Some people think you shouldn't fight the effects of ageing when it comes to sex: a woman should simply stop at menopause and a man should stop when he's no longer a 'stud'. Germain Greer has written that a woman might prefer to 'opt out' of sex at menopause if her partner 'takes a good deal longer about it' than he used to. Well, some women might. Nonetheless, as I hope I've demonstrated throughout this book, longer is better. And the emotional, intellectual and spiritual aspects of sex carry on regardless.

Insight
After the age of about 60, you may find that if you let your erection go down, you can't get it up again, even though you haven't ejaculated. If this is happening to you, the key is not to get erect until you're both ready for intercourse. In other words, concentrate on your partner and don't let her stimulate you. Just before intercourse, stimulate yourself or let your partner stimulate you with her mouth and fingers, enter your partner immediately and maintain a steady level of excitement.

Positions

There comes a time for everybody when they're just not as flexible (or as light) as they used to be. When that times comes, the following are pretty good positions. I've given the scores awarded by my focus groups (from one to 100) and left a space for you to add your own.

SPOONS

The woman simply lies on her side with her thighs approximately at right angles to her body and her knees bent. The man enters her from behind. A comfortable position for both.

Focus group score: 87   Your score: ....

THE IMPROVED MISSIONARY POSITION

The woman lies on the bed with sufficient pillows under her for the man to be able to kneel between her legs.

Focus group score: 86   Your score: ....

ON THE EDGE

The woman lies on the bed with her vulva at the edge and her legs hanging down. The man stands between her thighs. If the bed is too low, use pillows to raise her up. As a variation the woman can lie on her side.

Focus group score: 80   Your score: ....

PASSERS BY

The woman lies on her side, roughly in a banana shape. The man then enters from behind but upside down with his face close to her feet. This is a comfortable position for both, which makes it easy for the man to stimulate the woman's G-spot while she can stimulate her own clitoris.

Focus group score: 77   Your score: ....

THE CHAIR

The woman sits on a suitable chair and the man stands between her legs.

Focus group score: 75   Your score: ....

A lifetime of sex with the same partner

Is it possible to keep sex exciting right through a relationship that might last for 60 years or more? I believe it is.

It's important to keep finding new things to do, and I hope that this book has given you some fresh ideas. Most importantly, to stop looking at sex as a way of discharging 'lust' and look at it as a way of *creating*. As long as you have the creative impulse and creative ideas, you'll never be bored.

The research of Shere Hite and many others, as well as my focus groups, all confirm this. The comments of couples in their seventies and eighties are not only cause for optimism but are deeply moving. A man in his seventies has intercourse four or five times a week with a new partner, also in her seventies, who 'almost always has an orgasm'. A couple in their eighties who relish an hour of 'sex play' in the morning, a two-hour siesta 'naked in each other's arms' and another half hour or so of sex at night because every day is 'precious'. And the 82-year-old man who told me the greatest pleasure in sex was the feeling of 'oneness' with his wife.

Remember, you're not only having sex with a physical presence, you're having sex with a soul. Even if you don't literally believe that, you should at least reflect that the beauty of the inner person is by far the most important thing.

10 THINGS TO REMEMBER

1   *Sex can get better after the age of 50 for both women and men.*

2   *For women, the ratio of testosterone to oestrogen normally increases, thus boosting sex drive.*

3   *Every woman over 50 should have a vibrator, lots of lubricant and frequent sex.*

4   *There are food supplements that can help maintain physical and sexual form for both men and women.*

5   *Men over 50 should use erotica and masturbation without ejaculation to boost their testosterone levels.*

6   *Men over 50 can still have sex every day with multiple orgasms.*

7   *When multiple orgasms aren't possible, men over 50 can still have daily intercourse without orgasm or ejaculation.*

8   *The way of the Tao includes the philosophy that it's far more important to follow the road to ejaculation than to actually arrive.*

9   *As long as you're creative there are always new things you can find to do sexually.*

10 *There are couples in their eighties who still enjoy great sex.*

HOW GREAT IS SEX NOW?

▶ Is sex now better than when you were younger?   Yes/No

▶ Have you got at least one vibrator and are you
using it regularly?   Yes/No

▶ Are you using lubricant?   Yes/No

▶ Are you having some kind of sexual activity
most days?   Yes/No

▶ Are you making a deliberate effort to maintain your
libido by, for example, reading or watching erotica?   Yes/No

▶ Have you tried something new in sex this week?   Yes/No

▶ Are you able to masturbate in front of your partner
when you need more stimulation?   Yes/No

▶ Men: have you deliberately tried sex without either
orgasm or ejaculation?   Yes/No

If you answered 'no' to more than three questions, re-read the
relevant parts of the chapter and make an effort to put the
suggestions into effect. Sex can go on getting better and better even
into your seventies but only provided you make a conscious effort.
Don't respond to the years by having less sex, respond by having
different and more exciting sex. Decline is not inevitable. Bear in
mind that great results won't come from any one thing but from
the cumulative effect of all the different ideas together.

14

Great solutions to common sex problems

In this chapter you will learn:
- *how to solve some common sex problems for couples*
- *how to solve some common sex problems for men*
- *how to solve some common sex problems for women.*

Everyone faces problems with their sex lives from time to time. Fortunately, there is now a huge range of resources devoted to treating sexual dysfunction in all its forms, and a far greater understanding than ever before. Some problems can only be solved with professional help, but there are others you can deal with on your own.

Couples' problems

Sex, unfortunately, is a common cause of arguments between partners, particularly in the early years of a relationship.

If you're arguing about one specific thing to do with sex, then that problem is probably fairly easy to solve. However, if you find you're arguing about *everything* to do with sex then you are probably not sexually compatible. At least, not at the moment, but people do change over the years.

Communication is the first line of 'treatment'. Arguing is a form of communication, but not a very useful one. When you're both in a calm frame of mind set out your own positions. Don't make personal attacks and don't criticize. This will only make the other person defensive, resentful and less open to reason. Acknowledge that you understand your partner's point of view.

First, rid yourself of the notion (if you have it) that doing something to please your partner will somehow diminish you. If you're not particularly excited by something but don't have any particular objection to it, then why not just go along with it? If your man likes to see you in a suspender belt (but it gives you no pleasure), or your woman likes you to spend ten minutes massaging her (but it gives you no pleasure) then *do it* for him or her. That's called love. I guarantee that when one of you starts to put aside, let's call it 'pride', the other will start to do the same.

There are some things about sex (I stress *some*) about which you can say 'don't knock it if you haven't tried it'. Thus, someone may be convinced that, say, sex once a week is the ideal for him or her, but without ever having tried sex every day. Agree, if you can, that you'll try things your partner's way for an appropriate period, and that your partner will try things your way for an appropriate period. Then review things. You may find that there's no longer any argument. If there is, see if it's the kind of issue on which you can compromise.

There's another category of things about which you or your partner may hold such strong views that one of you is not even willing just to try. Anal sex is often such an issue. If you have a great sex life except for this one thing, then let it drop. If, for example, you're a man who wants your partner to try anal sex or fellatio to ejaculation, and she hates the idea, don't press it. There are so many, many techniques you can enjoy together that it's just not worth spoiling things over one. Hopefully, you're together for the long haul and, over time, people's attitudes can change. Could be yours. Could be your partner's. If you're really not getting anywhere, consider going together to a sex therapist.

Men's problems

SIZE

Many men are concerned about the size of their penises. Some think they're too small, while others (rather fewer) think they're too big.

As you saw in Chapter 3, the average size in erection is believed to be around 14 cm (5.5 inches). Nobody really knows. However, as you've also seen, the vagina is only around 7.5 cm (3 inches) long (in women who haven't had children), lengthening to 10 cm (4 inches) with sexual excitement. It actually has to stretch if a man's penis is longer than this. What's more, only the outer third of the vagina is very sensitive. Consequently, a woman certainly doesn't need a long penis to get excited. On the other hand, if her partner does have an unusually long penis he's going to have to use it with care.

It's often said that it's not the length of the penis that counts but what the man does with it. And it's true, it's simply a question of using different techniques.

For a shorter penis:

▶ *use positions that allow full insertion, such as the Ball and the Exhibitionist (pages 122–3)*
▶ *when thrusting, be careful not to slip out accidentally but, instead, slide out on purpose – women find it very exciting to be penetrated once and hugely exciting to be penetrated several times*

- ▶ *place love balls in the vagina, or a butt plug in the rectum – they can give a greater sense of fullness during intercourse.*

For a longer penis:

- ▶ *don't go for full insertion straight away; begin intercourse with only partial insertion and increase the depth gradually*
- ▶ *use positions that naturally inhibit full insertion such as the Rider, Autumn dog and the Improved missionary, variation 10 (pages 123, 133 and 119).*

Penis enlargement

Although it hasn't been 'scientifically proven', there's plenty of anecdotal evidence that a penis can be enlarged, without surgery. In the 1970s, Dr Brian Richards tested exercises and vacuum pumping on 32 men. Of those, 28 gained significant length (up to 4.9 cm/1.4 inches) as well as girth.

Nevertheless, it's very important to bear in mind that a penis is a very delicate piece of apparatus. *Never do anything that might harm your penis.* Damage could be permanent. In the USA, the Food and Drug Administration (FDA) has issued an alert about inadequate instructions with some mechanical penis enlargement products because all kinds of ruptures can result.

Rather than take a risk, I recommend you limit yourself to safe, gentle stretching and massage (known as 'jelqing'). It's a good idea to spread some suitable oil over your penis before you begin, just as you would for most kinds of massage. Evening primrose oil is the best because of the way it improves skin elasticity. Place your two thumbs on the side of the penis facing you and two or three fingers of each hand along the underside (but not pressing on the urethra). Now gently and slowly slide them along from the base to the glans. When you reach the tip, *gently* stretch out the penis by pulling on the foreskin (if you have one). Repeat. When you get an erection (in fact, this can be a good way of encouraging an erection), let it subside before continuing. Some men do this for a few minutes, some for up to 20 minutes. Don't expect immediate results, but over a period of months, at a minimum of three times a week, you *may* experience some enlargement. In any event, this gentle penis massage is beneficial to blood flow and, while you're at it, you may care to massage your testicles and perineum as well.

PREMATURE EJACULATION

Some sexologists define premature ejaculation as having an orgasm before you want to. Well, in that case, most men suffer from it! Another possible definition is the man having an orgasm before the woman wants him to. That is, before she's had at least one orgasm and possibly several. In practice, that's also very vague.

Perhaps, then, a time can be put to premature ejaculation? Back in Alfred Kinsey's day (as he demonstrated), most men ejaculated within two minutes of penetration on more than half the occasions they had sex. Since then, skills have improved. Typically, now, intercourse is thought to continue for about ten minutes.

Therefore, this question of 'premature' isn't as clear as it may seem. Quite probably, if you're worried that you're premature, you're no different to most other men. There are various ways in which you can delay ejaculation during intercourse:

▶ *Have sex more often.*
▶ *If you don't have a regular partner, or your regular partner doesn't want sex often enough, masturbate to ejaculation more frequently.*
▶ *When you masturbate, practise the control techniques described below and in Chapters 3 and 8.*
▶ *Wear a condom; if you already use condoms, select a thicker model.*
▶ *Smother your penis with silicone lubricant which will significantly reduce friction.*
▶ *Choose positions that provide less sensation, such as the Sitting embrace, variation 2 (page 124).*
▶ *Don't thrust, but while keeping your penis fully inserted, merely grind against her pelvic area.*

Remember that most women aren't interested in marathon intercourse. They can get sore or numb. It may be better to put more effort into what you do before intercourse and worry less about the length of intercourse itself.

Learning control
The first thing to fix very clearly in your mind is that the goal of sex is *not* ejaculation. After all, you'll inevitably ejaculate, unless you try very hard not to. So don't get fixated on it. The more quickly you ejaculate the more you deprive yourself of all the exquisite sensations that can only be enjoyed prior to ejaculation. Keep that in mind. What you want to do is revel in all the rapture that precedes ejaculation.

It could be that you have low serotonin (a chemical that cools down your sex drive). Try eating something sugary, say a few pieces of chocolate, a quarter of an hour before sex.

Get a clock (as suggested in Chapter 3) and put it in a prominent place. Determine that you'll masturbate for a specific length of time before you allow yourself to ejaculate. That length of time depends on your typical response – as a guide, begin by doubling the longest amount of time you've ever managed before.

The 'trick' is to learn to recognize the approach of the point of no return (PNR). Once you have a good erection, slow down and give yourself just enough stimulation to maintain it. Let's call this the base level. How does it feel? Enjoy the sensations without needing to intensify them. After a while, increase the stimulation a little and then let it die back to the base level again. Repeat this a few times. Now take the stimulation to a higher level and once again let it die back to the base level. Eventually you're going to get close to that PNR. You'll recognize it by a greater feeling of urgency and craving for orgasm. You'll probably feel things tensing up at the root of your penis. Don't give in. Immediately cease stimulation and, once again, let things die down. Quite probably some fluid will have escaped. This is helpful, because the more that seeps out without you actually ejaculating, the less urgent your desire for orgasm will be. Keep up this approaching and retreating from the PNR until the determined length of time has expired.

Basically, you can do exactly the same thing during intercourse by thrusting and then not thrusting. Of course, intercourse is far more complicated because of the extra stimulation provided by your partner who can also move. You'll have to agree a signal that means: 'Please don't move any more.' Holding your partner's hips still is probably the most convenient.

You may have to continue your masturbation 'homework' for a few weeks before things improve. Vary it by sometimes ending masturbation without ejaculation – just get on with something else and forget about it. While this 'training' is going on, also aim to discover the optimum frequency. For example, if you masturbate every other day does that make it easier to control ejaculation? Or does it have to be every day? Twice a day? Find out.

Naturally, if you can ejaculate a second time within a short while then the fact that your first orgasm was premature doesn't matter very much. The second won't be.

If none of this works, then, as a last resort, a doctor can prescribe pills that will help.

ERECTILE DYSFUNCTION

Most men suffer from erectile dysfunction at some time. There can be a whole variety of causes ranging from overwork through emotional stress to the use of certain medications.

William Masters and Virginia Johnson considered that erectile dysfunction was largely a psychological problem and, for many years, that was the prevailing view. Now, however, doctors consider it to be largely a physical problem.

To begin with, you might simply be trying to have ejaculatory sex too often. As you saw in Chapter 3, men need time for the body to become ready once again. As men get older, so this 'refractory' period gets longer and longer. If you try to have sex too soon, you may be capable of it – just – but it won't be with the same ease and vigour as it would be if you'd waited a while. Give yourself a little break. Check your responsiveness by masturbating (but don't ejaculate). Note that we're talking here about *ejaculatory* sex because it's principally (but not only) ejaculation that causes the refractory period. Switch to the techniques of multiple male orgasm (see Chapter 8) and the Tao (see Chapter 13) and you'll be making fewer demands on your body.

Just one failure to erect can lead to anxiety, and anxiety is the enemy of erection. As a result, it's vital that neither you nor your partner gets tense about it. Don't go staking all your masculinity on it. And think about her as well; she may feel that her femininity is under threat because she failed to excite you. Instead, both of you need to develop the mindset that if it happens it doesn't matter because there are still plenty of other things you can do. William Masters and Virginia Johnson developed a therapy which, basically, worked on this principle. Couples were told they could caress but that they couldn't have intercourse. Once the pressure was off in this way, a lot of men started to have erections again.

If you're not doing the PC muscle exercises in Chapter 11, get started right now. There's no question that they improve the circulation, increase erection and produce more vigorous orgasms. Also, have another look at the sex techniques described in Chapter 5. If you're not yet using some of the more powerful methods, then start trying them out; it's a fact of life that as you get older, so you need more stimulation. You may find the penis enlargement massage described above helps you to get an erection where normal friction doesn't. Man-on-top positions will be best simply because gravity will be helping the blood flow.

You may need to top up your testosterone and certain other chemicals. Your body's production of testosterone is not a constant; as men age, so production declines. Yet there are always things you can do to slow the decline and to give production a temporary nudge back up to the younger levels. Erotica will definitely give testosterone a boost. As you've seen, the enemies of testosterone and sex include:

▶ *alcohol*
▶ *tobacco*
▶ *a high fat intake*
▶ *a paunch*
▶ *lack of exercise.*

In Chapter 9, I said that I wouldn't recommend any herbs as aphrodisiacs because of the placebo effect and the risk of side effects. However, if you do have erectile dysfunction, that's a different situation and you might like to consider the following herbs, minerals and supplements:

▶ *Ginkgo biloba – its performance-enhancing effects are well-established in long-term use, probably by improving blood flow to erectile tissue (and also, it's suggested, in the brain).*
▶ *Nettle root – inhibits aromatase which, especially in men carrying a lot of fat, converts testosterone to the 'female' hormone oestrogen.*
▶ *Saw palmetto – helps to inhibit a chemical called 'sex hormone binding globulin' (SHBG) which, as it were, ties up testosterone in the body; the result is an increase in the all-important 'free' testosterone. It also inhibits enlargement of the prostate gland with age.*
▶ *Zinc – for reasons described in Chapter 11.*
▶ *Korean red ginseng and L-Arginine have both been scientifically proven to have at least some benefit in certain circumstances.*
▶ *Cistanchis, Cynomorium songaricum, Damiana, Epimedium sagittatum (horny goat weed), Eurycoma longfolia, Maca, Mucuna pruriens, Muira puama, Tribulus terrestris. There is plenty of anecdotal evidence that these are effective in various degrees.*

Food supplements take time to act. They don't have an almost instant effect like Viagra, so you'll have to take them over a period of weeks to see if they're having any effect on you. Remember that the controls over food supplements are not the same as those for medicines. Supplements sent for analysis often don't contain the claimed ingredients and sometimes contain toxins. Only buy from the most reputable sources you can find.

If the problem seems to be serious and long term, you should seek professional advice. Viagra is only the most famous of a whole range of treatments that are now available, and only a professional can decide what's right for you. Don't self-medicate with prescription drugs from the internet; drugs should *only* be prescribed by a doctor after a medical check-up.

If you prefer not to take 'drugs', a type of magnet therapy called pulsed electromagnetic field (PEMF) therapy may be for you. You have to wear a little box containing the apparatus close to the genitals.

Women's problems

FEMALE SEXUAL AROUSAL DISORDER

Women, sadly, have suffered a great deal at the hands of men. It's men, after all, who have defined what's 'normal' or 'abnormal' about a woman's sexual response. In the 1860s, Isaac Baker Brown wrote in his *Surgical Diseases of Women* that masturbation called for 'excision or amputation of the clitoris', and performed the operations at his London clinic. This was still being recommended in *The New System of Gynaecology* published in 1917. Sigmund Freud told women they were 'immature' if they had orgasms from clitoral stimulation. On that Freud was wrong. Now, some doctors in the USA are saying that about 45 per cent of women suffer from female sexual arousal disorder (FSAD), which is to say, an inability to become excited and have an orgasm. It's what used to be called 'frigidity'. But when almost half of all women are being labelled 'abnormal', it could be that the problem lies with men rather than women.

If you think there's something wrong with you; if you think your response isn't what it used to be; if you're not happy; or if you have a specific problem, then, of course, seek a solution. However, it's worth taking note of the feminists who say that *not* feeling desire for a dishevelled, unwashed, overweight and sexually incompetent companion is hardly a disorder. It's a good point; at least in some cases, FSAD might really be MUD – male unattractiveness disorder.

In general, women could be said to be sexually neutral. Unlike men, they usually need a good reason to feel aroused. So, guys, if your partner seems to you to be suffering from FSAD, just ask yourself if the problem doesn't lie with *you* rather than with her.

INABILITY TO ORGASM

The technical name for being unable to have an orgasm is 'anorgasmia'. There are various forms. If you've never had an orgasm it's 'primary anorgasmia'; if you've stopped being orgasmic it's 'secondary anorgasmia'; if you can have orgasms in some circumstances but not others it's 'situational anorgasmia'; if you can have orgasms but not from intercourse it's 'coital anorgasmia'; and if you have orgasms only now and then it's 'random anorgasmia'.

Many factors can affect a woman's ability to orgasm with a partner, including his skill and attractiveness to her, the situation, the degree of privacy, and the time available. If you orgasm during private masturbation, then it's obviously not a physical problem. Just as with men, anxiety (about other things as well as sex) affects performance. If, after trying all the techniques in this book, you still can't orgasm, you should consult a doctor and consider sex therapy.

PAIN

A tiny proportion of women suffer vaginismus in which the muscles around the entrance to the vagina go into *involuntary* spasms, thus preventing intercourse. I stress the word 'involuntary' because many of these women enjoy everything else about sex and want penetration. In the milder form, intercourse is possible but painful. There are other varied causes of pain (dyspareunia) which can come at any stage of intercourse and take the form of burning, sharp or cramping sensations. All of these conditions call for professional help.

DRYNESS

Dryness is easily dealt with. Simply buy a good quality lubricant from the chemist or sex shop and don't give the subject another thought (unless the dryness is severe and in combination with other problems of menopause). Remember that only water-based or silicone lubricants can be used with latex condoms, never oil-based types. If you have reached the menopause, read the section below on hormone replacement therapy (HRT).

NOISY VAGINA

Many women are embarrassed when their vagina makes a noise. In fact, it's entirely normal. So normal, in fact, that there are even recognized slang words for it – a 'vart' or, in more common usage, a 'queef'. The noise is due to the escape of air that has been pumped in by a man's thrusting. It happens mostly in rear-entry positions. There's nothing that can be done to prevent it entirely, but shorter thrusts and a change of angle will help. Occasionally, air trapped in the vagina can be uncomfortable or even painful. If that happens to you, ask your man to disengage and then resume after a moment in a face-to-face position. All men know about this, unless they're very inexperienced, so there's really no need to worry about it.

THE MENOPAUSE AND HORMONE REPLACEMENT THERAPY

Some women have no problems at all with the menopause, while others suffer fairly severe symptoms. For women who do have symptoms, they normally last from six months to two years, but hot flushes can continue for five years or more. Of course, changes like thinning of the vaginal walls and a reduction in lubrication continue indefinitely. Women's personalities can also change for a time; in particular, they may get angry very easily, when they never did before.

Hormone replacement therapy (HRT) can alleviate some symptoms by boosting oestrogen, the 'female' hormone that declines at the menopause. Progestogen is included in some forms of HRT to protect against cancer of the uterus. Yet another type increases testosterone (see below). Many women are very happy with HRT but there is an increased risk of breast cancer. How significant is it? For postmenopausal women aged 50–65:

▶ *of those not on HRT, around 32 in 1,000 will get breast cancer*
▶ *of those on oestrogen-only HRT for ten years, around 37 will get breast cancer*
▶ *of those on oestrogen-progestogen HRT for ten years, around 51 will get breast cancer.*

The increased risk is fairly small, and all the more so if HRT is only used for a year or two.

Before embarking on HRT, it's certainly worth trying herbal remedies (highly rated by many women). There's good evidence for Ginkgo biloba and anecdotal evidence for Damiana, Maca, Muira puama and Tribulus terrestris. Include soya, linseed, alfalfa and mung beans in your diet because they are all high in oestrogen-like substances known as 'phyto-oestrogens'. Regular sex (using lubricants) is also beneficial. However, if none of this helps then the decision about whether or not to try HRT is only one you can take in conjunction with a qualified professional. HRT can take various forms, including tablets, patches, implants, sprays and creams.

Testosterone replacement
As you've seen, women also have the 'male' hormone testosterone. It works just the same as it does in men's bodies to maintain muscles, strengthen bones, boost libido and increase the sensitivity of the genitals and nipples. As with men, testosterone in women

declines with age, and at 40 the level may be only half what it was at 20. Testosterone replacement is relatively new; it certainly works for a lot of women but the long-term effects aren't known. An alternative is to take DHEA, the precursor to testosterone, but this should only be done under medical supervision because of possible side effects. Allow about four months to see if it will work for you.

Sexually transmitted diseases

When you begin a new sexual relationship, you run the risk of contracting a sexually transmitted disease (STD) (just as you do if an existing partner sleeps with anyone else, of course). It doesn't matter how attractive or nice the new person in your life is. Diseases don't discriminate over things like that; anybody can contract an STD. It is as likely to happen the first time you ever have sex in your life as it is the thousandth time. (In fact, statistically, young people are *more* likely to be infected than older people.)

The new person in your life will also be wondering about his or her chances of contracting an STD from you. So, there's no need to be hesitant about discussing the subject *before* you get into bed.

Try to find out about your prospective partner's sexual history. Yet even if he or she has been sexually inactive for a while, the first unbreakable rule is that you must use condoms. How long you continue to use them depends on several factors. Be aware that the HIV antibody test does not give a reliable result for approximately the first three months, and that chlamydia can be invisible.

If you're already using the pill or some other form of contraception, you don't have to *say* you are. Insist on a condom being used. A man with any sense would want to use a condom for his own protection, anyway. If he refuses, don't have sex with him.

Syphilis
▶ Route of infection. *Intercourse, genital contact with mouth, fingers, etc., blood transfusion, mother to foetus.*

- ▶ How to recognize the symptoms. *Two to four weeks after sexual contact a sore known as a 'chancre' appears as a spot which then ulcerates. Chancres are most common on the genitals and anus but can also be on the lips, mouth, fingers or breasts. One to 26 weeks after the chancre heals there can be a rash, fever, sore throat, headaches, joint pains, loss of appetite and hair loss; infectious moist sores appear around the genitals and anus.*
- ▶ Is it serious? *Very. Years later syphilis can cause heart, eye, brain and spinal cord damage leading to blindness, paralysis, insanity and death.*

Gonorrhea

- ▶ Route of infection. *Any sexual contact including, in rare cases, kissing.*
- ▶ How to recognize the symptoms. *Two to 30 days after sexual contact men develop a yellow discharge from the penis, while women develop vaginal discharge, irritation of the genitals and a burning pain on urinating.*
- ▶ Is it serious? *Yes. In both sexes it may lead to sterility if untreated.*

Acquired Immune Deficiency Syndrome (AIDS)

- ▶ Route of infection. *Begins with transmission of the HIV virus by vaginal or anal intercourse without a condom; the use of a condom significantly reduces the risk. Oral sex and deep kissing have, in rare cases, also led to HIV transmission.*
- ▶ How to recognize the symptoms. *After infection some people have no symptoms at first, but within three to six weeks others have flu-like symptoms (Acute HIV Syndrome) including fever, headache, nausea, diarrhoea and enlargement of the lymph nodes. After these have cleared up, victims may be clear of symptoms for months or years but then develop weight loss, thrush, fevers, extreme fatigue, diarrhoea, coughing, shortness of breath, rashes, discoloured growths on the skin or inside the mouth, numbness and other problems.*
- ▶ Is it serious? *Yes. Once the HIV virus is inside the body it will eventually lead to the development of AIDS. As yet, there is no*

cure although 'highly active antiretroviral therapy' (HAART) has significantly reduced AIDS-related deaths.

Human papillomavirus (HPV)

- ▶ Route of infection. *Skin to skin contact during sex.*
- ▶ How to recognize the symptoms. *In some strains of the virus, cauliflower-like growths in moist areas around the sex organs; other strains may eventually lead to cancer.*
- ▶ Is it serious? *The warts can be removed and the virus that caused them will normally reduce to undetectable levels, although in some cases victims may remain contagious. The dangerous strains are those that don't cause warts but may eventually lead to cancer of the cervix, vulva, penis or anus.*

Genital herpes

- ▶ Route of infection. *Genital contact.*
- ▶ How to recognize the symptoms. *Clusters of small blisters appear on the genitals and later burst to form ulcers, which heal within one to three weeks. However, the virus invades the nerves in the pelvic region and can cause renewed attacks. Victims should not have sex for two weeks after the sores have completely healed, but even then a risk to their partners remains.*
- ▶ Is it serious? *It increases the risk that genital warts will cause cervical cancer; potentially very serious for a foetus.*

Chlamydia

- ▶ Route of infection. *Vaginal, anal or oral sex.*
- ▶ How to recognize the symptoms. *One to three weeks after exposure women may have vaginal discharge and burning when urinating; later there may be pain during intercourse, bleeding, back pain, abdominal pain, fever and nausea. Men may have burning and itching around the opening of the penis; rarely, there's swelling of the testicles.*
- ▶ Is it serious? *In women, if untreated, it can lead to sterility, pelvic pain and an increased risk of pregnancy outside the uterus as well as an increased risk of contracting the HIV virus if exposed. In men, infection can spread to the tube that carries sperm from the testicles.*

Non-specific urethritis

▶ Route of infection. *Unprotected sex.*

▶ How to recognize the symptoms. *Pain on urination or during sex. Cloudy white or yellow-green discharge from the penis.*

▶ Is it serious? *Antibiotics can cure it.*

HOW SAFE ARE CONDOMS?

Condoms are recommended during the first six months of a relationship. But how safe are they in preventing the transmission of STDs? The Centers for Disease Control and Prevention in the USA has concluded that latex condoms provide an essentially impermeable barrier to particles the size of STD pathogens. However, the level of protection varies depending on whether *discharge* diseases or *contact* diseases are involved. Discharge diseases are those in which the infection is transmitted by infected semen or vaginal fluid, and include HIV, gonorrhea and chlamydia. Contact diseases are those in which the infection is spread by contact with infected skin or mucosal surfaces and for which, therefore, condoms may be of limited use; they include genital herpes, syphilis and genital warts.

Table 4 How effective are condoms?

Disease	Route of transmission	Centers for Disease Control and Prevention assessment
HIV	Discharge diseases	Highly effective
Gonorrhea, Chlamydia	Discharge diseases	Reduce the risk
Herpes, Syphilis, HPV	Contact diseases	Reduce the risk*

*Provided the affected area is covered by the condom.

10 THINGS TO REMEMBER

1 Communication, in a calm atmosphere, is always the first 'treatment' for disagreements about sex.

2 Don't spoil a great relationship by insisting on a technique your partner doesn't like.

3 Penis size is rarely a problem – there are techniques for all sizes; if you're really concerned, penis enlargement may be possible by jelqing.

4 Premature ejaculation can usually be controlled by practising special techniques; medication is available as a last resort.

5 Erectile dysfunction can often be treated simply by removing the pressure to ejaculate; don't self-medicate with prescription drugs from the internet.

6 Female sexual arousal disorder (FSAD) may often be more accurately called male unattractiveness disorder (MUD) or simply be due to anxiety.

7 Treat symptoms of the menopause the 'natural' way before considering hormone replacement therapy (HRT).

8 Just as much as it is to men, testosterone is important to women and can be supplemented; the hormone DHEA may help if given under medical supervision.

9 When beginning a new relationship, it's important for you both to be frank about your sexual histories; if there's any doubt, testing is essential.

10 Always use condoms for at least the first six months of a new relationship; when properly used, they offer a high degree of protection against HIV transmission.

HOW GREAT IS SEX NOW?

▶ *Are you happily discussing and planning your sex life together?*   Yes/No

▶ *Are you willing to do things simply to pleasure your partner even though they give no particular pleasure to you?*   Yes/No

▶ *Men: have you given up worrying about the size of your penis?*   Yes/No

▶ *Men: are you giving your penis a regular jelqing?*   Yes/No

▶ *Men: if you've been suffering from premature ejaculation, have you followed the advice?*   Yes/No

▶ *Men: if you've been suffering from erectile dysfunction, have you followed the advice?*   Yes/No

▶ *Women: if your libido is down, have you determined whether it's FSAD or MUD?*   Yes/No

▶ *Women: if it's FSAD, are you following all the advice in this book to boost libido?*   Yes/No

▶ *Women: if you're having problems with the menopause, have you tried regular sex (with lubricants) as a form of treatment?*   Yes/No

▶ *Men and women: if you're dating, are you using condoms?*   Yes/No

If you answered 'no' to more than three relevant questions, re-read the relevant parts of the chapter and make an effort to put the suggestions into effect. Most sex problems can be fixed fairly easily if you can discuss things frankly with your partner and are willing to make some lifestyle changes. For more intractable problems, don't be afraid to seek professional help.

Taking it further

The Art of Loving, Erich Fromm, Thorsons, 1957

The Change, Germaine Greer, Hamish Hamilton, 1991

Emotional Intelligence, Daniel Goleman, Bloomsbury, 1996

The ESO Ecstasy Program: Better, Safer Sexual Intimacy and Extended Orgasmic Response, Alan Brauer and Donna Brauer, Warner Books, 1990

Eve's Secrets: A New Theory of Female Sexuality, J. L. Sevely, Random House, 1987

Exotic Massage for Lovers, Timothy Freke, Eddison Sadd Edition, 1996

Female Ejaculation & The G-Spot, Deborah Sundahl, Fusion Press, 2004

Food Pharmacy, Jean Carper, Simon & Schuster, 1989

Get Intimate with Tantric Sex, Paul Jenner, Hodder Education, 2010

The G-Spot and Other Discoveries about Human Sexuality, Alice Ladas, Beverly Whipple and John Perry, Holt, Rinehart and Winston, 1982

The Hite Report on Male Sexuality, Shere Hite, Ballantine Books, 1981

Human Sexuality, William Masters and Virginia Johnson, Little Brown, 1982

Human Sexual Response, William Masters and Virginia Johnson, Little Brown, 1966/Bantam, 1980

Intimate Touch, Michael Reed Gach, Piatkus, 1997

The Joy of Sexual Fantasy, Dr Andrew Stanway, Headline, 1991

Multi-Orgasmic Couple, Mantak Chia, Maneewan Chia, Douglas Abrams and Rachel Carlton Abrams M.D., Thorsons, 2000

The Multi-Orgasmic Man, Mantak Chia and Douglas Abrams Arava, Thorsons, 2001

The New Hite Report, Shere Hite, Hamlyn, 1976

The Pocket Book of Foreplay, Richard Craze, Hunter House Books, 2000

The Pocket Book of Sexual Fantasies, Richard Craze, Hunter House Books, 2000

The Science of Love, Anthony Walsh, Ph.D, Prometheus Books, 1996

Simultaneous Orgasm, Michael Riskin and Anita Banker-Riskin, Hunter House Books, 1997

The Surrender, Toni Bentley, Harper Collins, 2004.

The Tao of Love, Jolan Chang, Wildwood House Ltd, 1977

You Just Don't Understand, Deborah Tannen, Virago Press, 1991

Courses

MASSAGE COURSES

www.massagefree.com
www.tantra.com

SEX COURSES

www.eroticuniversity.com

STRIPTEASE COURSES

UK
www.jumpanddance.com
www.londonschoolofstriptease.co.uk

USA
www.urbanstriptease.com

Sex counselling

UK
www.basrt.org.uk – The British Association for Sexual and Relationship Therapy.

www.brook.org.uk – Sexual health advice, contraception and counselling for those aged 25 and under.
www.ipm.org.uk – The Institute of Psychosexual Medicine.
www.relate.org.uk – Modestly priced help with sex and relationships.

USA
www.aasect.org – The American Association of Sexuality.
www.councilforrelationships.org
www.sexualtherapy.com – The Institute for Marital and Sexual Therapy.

Sex and the internet

Exercise extreme caution when surfing the internet for information and/or products to do with sex. You could find yourself, quite inadvertently, looking at material that is illegal and morally indefensible. All the sites listed here have a serious intent.

The author has his own website at www.pauljenner.eu and will be happy to receive your feedback.

CONTRACEPTION

UK
www.brook.org.uk
www.netdoctor.co.uk
www.thesite.org
www.spired.com

USA
www.avert.org
www.choose-health.com
http://dmoz.org/health/reproductive_health

INTERNET SHOPPING

UK

www.passion8.co.uk – A reliable UK supplier with a wide range of sex toys, lingerie, lubricants and erotica.

www.coco-de-mer-shop.com – The mail order department of the elegant Covent Garden shop selling luxurious jade dildos, edible massage oils, body jewellery, whips and, in fact, everything for wealthy lovers.

www.sextoys.co.uk

www.bedroompleasures.co.uk

www.lovehoney.co.uk

USA

http://store.sextoys.sex-superstore.com

www.toyssexshop.com

HOW SEX WORKS

www.arhp.org – The site for the Association of Reproductive Health Professionals.

www.healthyplace.com/sex/menu-id-66

SEX TECHNIQUES

http://dodsonandross.com

www.ivillage.co.uk/relationships/sex

http://sexuality.about.com

www.sexuality.org

www.take-it-like-a-man.com

Masturbation

http://advancedmasturbation.com (male only)

www.mymasturbation.com

http://sexuality.about.com/od/masturbation

SEXUAL HEALTH

www.bupa.co.uk
www.cdc.gov/std/healthcomm/fact_sheets.htm
http://health.discovery.com
www.healthsquare.com
www.sexualwellness.org
www.youandaids.org
www.avert.org

SEX FUN

www.world-sex-records.com
www.mysexgames.com

SEX DURING PREGNANCY

http://kidshealth.org/parent/pregnancy_newborn/pregnancy/sex_
  pregnancy.html
www.netdoctor.co.uk

SEX OVER 50

www.hellsgeriatrics.co.uk
www.letlifein.com
www.senior-center.com/sexlife.htm

The publisher has used its best endeavours to ensure that the URLs for external websites referred to in this book are correct and active at the time of going to press. However, the publisher and the author have no responsibility for the websites and can make no guarantee that a site will remain live or that the content will remain relevant, decent or appropriate.

Index

Image credits